T0226664

Ultrasound: Part 2

Editor

TERESA S. WU

CRITICAL CARE CLINICS

www.criticalcare.theclinics.com

Consulting Editor
RICHARD W. CARLSON

April 2014 • Volume 30 • Number 2

ELSEVIER

1600 John F. Kennedy Boulevard • Suite 1800 • Philadelphia, Pennsylvania, 19103-2899

http://www.theclinics.com

CRITICAL CARE CLINICS Volume 30, Number 2
April 2014 ISSN 0749-0704, ISBN-13: 978-0-323-28993-1

Editor: Patrick Manley
Developmental Editor: Casey Jackson

Critical Care Clinics (ISSN: 0749-0704) is published quarterly by Elsevier Inc., 360 Park Avenue South, New York, NY 10010-1710. Months of issue are January, April, July, and October. Business and Editorial Offices: 1600 John F. Kennedy Blvd., Suite 1800, Philadelphia, PA 19103-2899. Customer Service Office: 6277 Sea Harbor Drive, Orlando, FL 32887-4800. Periodicals postage paid at New York, NY and additional mailing offices. Subscription prices are $210.00 per year for US individuals, $503.00 per year for US institution, $100.00 per year for US students and residents, $255.00 per year for Canadian individuals, $630.00 per year for Canadian institutions, $300.00 per year for international individuals, $630.00 per year for international institutions and $150.00 per year for Canadian and foreign students/residents. To receive student/resident rate, orders must be accompanied by name of affiliated institution, date of term, and the signature of program/residency coordinator on institution letterhead. Orders will be billed at individual rate until proof of status is received. Foreign air speed delivery is included in all *Clinics* subscription prices. All prices are subject to change without notice. POSTMASTER: Send address changes to *Critical Care Clinics*, Elsevier Periodicals Customer Service, 11830 Westline Industrial Drive, St. Louis, MO 63146. **Customer Service: 1-800-654-2452 (US). From outside of the US, call 1-314-447-8871. Fax: 1-314-447-8029. E-mail: journalscustomerservice-usa@ elsevier.com (for print support) or journalsonlinesupport-usa@elsevier.com (for online support).**

Reprints. For copies of 100 or more of articles in this publication, please contact the Commercial Reprints Department, Elsevier Inc., 360 Park Avenue South, New York, NY 10010-1710. Tel.: 212-633-3874; Fax: 212-633-3820; E-mail: reprints@elsevier.com.

Critical Care Clinics is also published in Spanish by Editorial Inter-Medica, Junin 917, 1ᵉʳ A, 1113, Buenos Aires, Argentina.

Critical Care Clinics is covered in *MEDLINE/PubMed (Index Medicus), EMBASE/Excerpta Medica, Current Concepts/ Clinical Medicine, ISI/BIOMED, and Chemical Abstracts.*

Printed and bound by CPI Group (UK) Ltd, Croydon, CR0 4YY

Contributors

CONSULTING EDITOR

RICHARD W. CARLSON, MD, PhD
Chairman Emeritus, Director, Medical Intensive Care Unit, Department of Medicine, Maricopa Medical Center; Professor, University of Arizona College of Medicine; Professor, Department of Medicine, Mayo Graduate School of Medicine, Phoenix, Arizona

EDITOR

TERESA S. WU, MD, FACEP
Director, Emergency Medicine Ultrasound Program and Fellowship; Co-Director, Simulation Based Training Program and Fellowship; Associate Program Director, Emergency Medicine Residency Program; Associate Professor, Department of Emergency Medicine, Maricopa Medical Center, Maricopa Integrated Health Care System, University of Arizona College of Medicine-Phoenix, Phoenix, Arizona

AUTHORS

CALEB BARR, MD
Department of Emergency Medicine, Palmetto Health Richland, Columbia, South Carolina

LAUREL BARR, MD
Emergency Medicine Resident, Department of Emergency Medicine, Maricopa Medical Center, Phoenix, Arizona

JUSTIN BOSLEY, MD
Resident, Department of Emergency Medicine, Highland Hospital, Alameda County Medical Center, Oakland, California

MARY J. CONNELL, MD
Ultrasound Section Chief, Maricopa Integrated Health Care System; Program Director, Diagnostic Radiology Residency, Maricopa Medical Center; Associate Professor of Radiology, Radiology Clerkship Director, University of Arizona College of Medicine-Phoenix, Phoenix, Arizona

THOMAS COOK, MD
Department of Emergency Medicine, Palmetto Health Richland, Columbia, South Carolina

NICHOLAS HATCH, MD
Emergency Medicine Resident, Department of Emergency Medicine, Medical Illustrator, Maricopa Medical Center, Phoenix, Arizona

PATRICK HUNT, MD
Department of Emergency Medicine, Palmetto Health Richland, Columbia, South Carolina

JACOB C. MISS, MD
Ultrasound Fellow, Department of Emergency Medicine, Highland Hospital, Alameda
County Medical Center, Oakland, California

LAURA NOLTING, MD
Department of Emergency Medicine, Palmetto Health Richland, Columbia,
South Carolina

PEDRO J. ROQUE, MD
Emergency Medicine Resident, Department of Emergency Medicine, Maricopa Medical
Center, Phoenix, Arizona

APARAJITA SOHONI, MD
Director of Medical Student Education/Attending Physician, Department of Emergency
Medicine, Highland Hospital, Alameda County Medical Center, Oakland, California

TERESA S. WU, MD, FACEP
Director, Emergency Medicine Ultrasound Program and Fellowship; Co-Director,
Simulation Based Training Program and Fellowship; Associate Program Director,
Emergency Medicine Residency Program; Associate Professor, Department of
Emergency Medicine, Maricopa Medical Center, Maricopa Integrated Health Care
System, University of Arizona College of Medicine-Phoenix, Phoenix, Arizona

Contents

Use of bedside ultrasound to guide simple procedures increases safety by allowing real-time visualization of patient anatomy. This article discusses ultrasound guidance for basic procedures including peripheral and central intravenous access, arterial access, suprapubic aspiration, abscess incision and drainage, foreign body identification, and joint arthrocentesis. It reviews the indications and complications of the procedure, advantages of ultrasound guidance, anatomy, and procedural technique.

Ultrasound guidance has become the standard of care for many bedside procedures, owing to its portability, ease of use, and significant reduction in complications. This article serves as an introduction to the use of ultrasonography in several advanced procedures, including pericardiocentesis, thoracentesis, paracentesis, lumbar puncture, regional anesthesia, and peritonsillar abscess drainage.

CRITICAL CARE CLINICS

Diagnostic Ultrasonography for Peripheral Vascular Emergencies

Thomas Cook, MD, Laura Nolting, MD*, Caleb Barr, MD,
Patrick Hunt, MD

KEYWORDS

- Ultrasonography • Deep vein thrombosis • Arterial occlusion • Pseudoaneurysm
- Aneurysm

KEY POINTS

- This article discusses how to differentiate the arterial from the venous system by ultrasonography, using real-time scanning, color Doppler, and pulsed-wave Doppler.
- This article describes the approach to detecting deep vein thrombosis in the acute care setting.
- Peripheral arterial aneurysm can present clinically as an asymptomatic pulsatile mass or acute limb-threatening ischemia. This article discusses the detection of peripheral aneurysms using ultrasonography.
- Pseudoaneurysms, while rare, do occur in the acute care setting. This article describes the ultrasonographic findings of pseudoaneurysm, and detection by ultrasonography of acute arterial occlusion.

INTRODUCTION

Regardless of whether an extremity is swollen, painful, tender, cool, pulseless, or possesses an enlarged mass, it is often caused by vascular abnormality. The bedside evaluation of peripheral vascular emergencies now relies on diagnostic ultrasonography more than any other laboratory or imaging modality. Having the skills to perform ultrasonography at the bedside not only expedites the care of seriously ill patients but also provides the clinician-sonographer the ability to examine other areas of the body that might be affected by acute disease of the peripheral vasculature.

C. Barr has identified no professional or financial affiliations for himself or his spouse/partner. These authors have identified a professional affiliation for themselves: T. Cook and P. Hunt are founders of 3rd Rock Ultrasound, LLC. 3rd Rock Ultrasound has agreements with the following companies to provide equipment and support to the ultrasound course: Sonosite, Siemens, Philips, Mindray, Terason, and GE. L. Nolting is an instructor for 3rd Rock Ultrasound, LLC.
Department of Emergency Medicine, Palmetto Health Richland, 14 Medical Park, Suite 350, Columbia, SC 29203, USA
* Corresponding author.
E-mail address: lanolting@gmail.com

Crit Care Clin 30 (2014) 185–206
http://dx.doi.org/10.1016/j.ccc.2013.10.006
0749-0704/14/$ – see front matter © 2014 Elsevier Inc. All rights reserved.

This article provides information needed for the use of ultrasonography in the diagnosis of emergent pathology of the peripheral vasculature. It covers the sonographic evaluation of deep vein thrombosis (DVT) and the peripheral arterial emergencies of aneurysm, pseudoaneurysm, and obstruction. Techniques and anatomy related to performing and interpreting these ultrasonography studies are emphasized. Aortic aneurysms and ultrasound-guided vascular access are discussed in another article elsewhere in this issue.

TECHNICAL CONSIDERATIONS OF PERIPHERAL VASCULAR SONOGRAPHY
Transducer Selection

Because peripheral vascular structures are relatively small and superficial, high-resolution ultrasound transducers are required. Linear-array, high-frequency transducers provide the best 2-dimensional image resolution, and are therefore preferred for these sonographic examinations (**Fig. 1**).

Color Doppler Ultrasonography

Even relatively inexpensive systems now have Doppler ultrasound capability. Color Doppler ultrasound technology uses the change in frequencies caused by blood flow to create corresponding images on the viewing screen. If the blood flow is moving toward the transducer, the return echo will have a higher frequency than was originally generated by the ultrasound system. When this occurs the ultrasound system will, by default, create a red image on the screen that represents the moving blood. If the blood flow is moving away from the transducer, the return echo will have a lower frequency than was originally generated by the ultrasound system. When this occurs, the ultrasound system will create a blue image on the screen (**Fig. 2**). With all Doppler imaging, the brighter the color, the faster the blood is moving. Color Doppler imaging only occurs within a relatively small area of the viewing screen referred to as the region of interest.

It is imperative for the clinician-sonographer to be correctly oriented to the vasculature. Typically the transducer should be oriented so that arterial flow is moving toward the probe and venous flow is moving away. If this is done, arterial blood flow will appear red and venous blood flow will appear blue. If the transducer is oriented so that the venous flow is moving toward the transducer, the color of arterial and venous blood will be reversed.

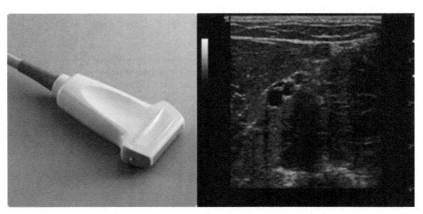

Fig. 1. Linear-array transducer with image of upper extremity vasculature.

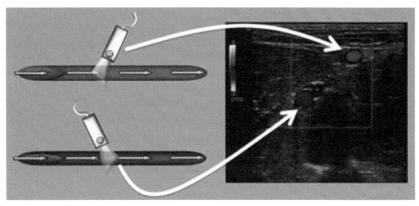

Fig. 2. Blood flow toward the transducer is red. Blood flow away from the transducer is blue. Doppler images are only seen within the rectangular box on the viewing screen. This area is referred to as the region of interest.

In addition, the ultrasound signal should be directed as close to parallel as possible to the flow of blood. When the ultrasound signal is perpendicular to the flow of blood, the ultrasound system cannot give accurate information regarding the direction and velocity of the moving blood (**Fig. 3**).

Pulsed-Wave Doppler Ultrasonography

Pulsed-wave Doppler (PWD) systems are able to provide Doppler shift data from a small segment along the ultrasound beam referred to as the sample volume or sample gate. The machine operator controls the location of this segment (**Fig. 4**).

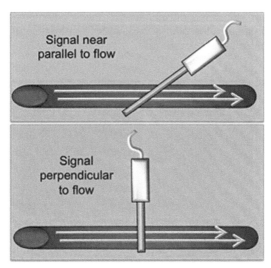

Fig. 3. To obtain accurate data using Doppler ultrasonography, the examiner needs to orient the ultrasound signal as close to parallel as possible to the flow of blood (*top*). If the ultrasound signal is perpendicular to the blood flow (*bottom*), Doppler ultrasonography cannot be used accurately.

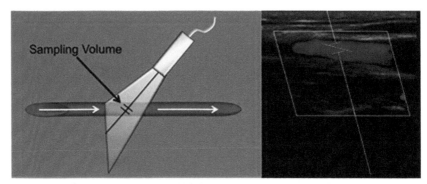

Fig. 4. With pulsed-wave Doppler (PWD) the examiner places a sample volume to measure the flow characteristics of blood.

PWD converts the measured change in frequencies caused by blood flow within the sample volume into audible sounds or visual data graphed over time. With the audible sounds, higher-pitched sounds are the result of higher Doppler shifts, and thus indicate higher flow rates. Lower-pitched sounds are from lower Doppler shifts caused by lower flow rates. Interpretation of these sounds is more subjective, but the difference in flow rates is fairly easy to distinguish.

When PWD converts blood-flow data into a visual display, the characteristics of the blood flowing at the sample volume are graphed over time (**Fig. 5**). A baseline indicating no flow is seen on the viewing screen. If blood is flowing toward the transducer, a waveform will be seen above a baseline. If the blood is flowing away from the transducer, a waveform will be seen below the baseline.

Comparison of Arterial and Venous Ultrasound Findings

With 2-dimensional ultrasonography, arteries will be pulsatile and have thicker walls than veins; however, it is often difficult to see these differences when examining smaller vessels. Fortunately, there are 4 techniques that can be used to differentiate peripheral arteries from veins (**Box 1**).

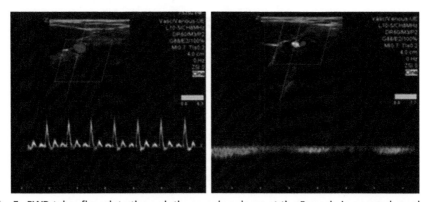

Fig. 5. PWD takes flow data through the sample volume at the B-mode image and graphs it over time at the bottom. The waveform on the left indicates that blood is flowing toward the transducer. The waveform on the right indicates that blood is flowing away from the transducer.

Box 1
Techniques for differentiating vessels
Compression
Doppler color flow
Pulsed-wave Doppler
Distal augmentation

Compression is the most commonly used technique. Veins are much more compliant then arteries and normally can be completely compressed with light pressure, whereas arteries remain patent until a greater amount of pressure is applied.

Doppler color flow can be used to demonstrate the direction of blood flow and the presence or absence of arterial pulsations. Color flow can also be used to determine whether a given structure is nonvascular. Examples of this include lymph nodes, abscesses, cysts (ie, Baker cyst at the popliteal fossa), seromas, and hematomas.

PWD can differentiate arteries from veins by examination of the waveform created by the flow of blood at the sample volume. Arterial blood flow is pulsatile, whereas normal venous flow is continuous without evidence of pulsations (**Fig. 6**).

Distal augmentation is another technique for identifying veins and the presence of venous obstruction. While using Doppler, the examiner gently compresses the vessel distal to the placement of the transducer. If the vessel on the viewing screen is a patent vein, the compression of the vein distally will result in a momentary increase in blood flow at the transducer site (**Fig. 7**).

DEEP VEIN THROMBOSIS

German physician Rudolph Virchow (1821–1902) was the first person to postulate the processes resulting in venous thrombosis during the nineteenth century, and his triad is still taught today (**Box 2**). Based on this triad, a list of risk factors for DVT can be generated (**Box 3**).

Wells Criteria

Before laboratory testing or imaging for the presence of DVT, the pretest probability should be determined using the Wells criteria (**Table 1**).[1]

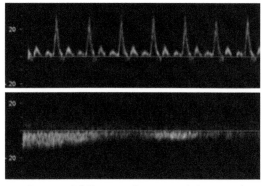

Fig. 6. PWD demonstrating arterial flow moving toward the transducer (*top*), and venous blood flow moving away from the transducer (*bottom*).

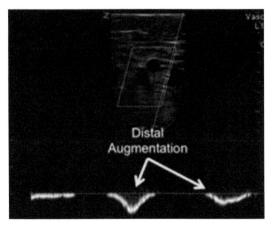

Fig. 7. PWD demonstrating venous distal augmentation.

Based on the total score obtained from the application of the Wells criteria, patients can be stratified into groups of low, moderate, and high probability (**Table 2**).

D-Dimer

D-dimer is a fibrin degradation product that is present in the blood after a blood clot is degraded by fibrinolysis. The test has significant clinical use in the evaluation of a patient for DVT. Of the different tests available to measure D-dimer, the enzyme-linked immunosorbent assay is the most sensitive (>95%), and a negative test result can practically rule out thromboembolism in patients with a low pretest probability of DVT. However, all tests for D-dimer are not specific, so a positive result does not mean that thromboembolism is present.

DVT Evaluation Algorithm

The Wells criteria, in combination with a sensitive D-dimer assay, can be effectively used in an algorithm for the evaluation of a patient for DVT (**Fig. 8**). If the score generated by the Wells criteria places the patient in the High-Probability category, the patient should undergo ultrasonography evaluation regardless of the result of the D-dimer. If the patient does not have DVT by ultrasonography but is stratified in the High-Probability category, a repeat sonogram in 1 week should be considered.[2]

Ultrasonography Findings of DVT

The diagnosis of DVT by ultrasonography is accomplished by identifying 1 or more of the findings listed in **Box 4**.

Of these 4 findings, the most helpful to the examiner is the inability to completely compress the lumen of the vein with the ultrasound transducer (**Fig. 9**).[3] The low

| Box 2 |
| Virchow's triad |
| Stasis of blood flow |
| Endothelial injury |
| Hypercoagulable state |

Box 3
Risk factors for deep vein thrombosis
Increasing age
Surgery
Cancer
Trauma
Immobility
Estrogen therapy
Pregnancy and the postpartum period
Indwelling intravenous catheters

intraluminal pressure in addition to the thin vessel wall of veins makes them very easy to compress relative to adjacent arteries. If the examiner cannot achieve complete apposition of the superficial and deep wall of the vein with compression ultrasound (CUS), there must be something in the vessel lumen preventing this from occurring (and this is almost always a thrombus).

The presence of intraluminal echogenic material from a venous thrombus is also often seen on examination, but is not required to make the diagnosis (**Fig. 10**) of DVT. Acute thrombus is less likely than chronic thrombus to demonstrate echogenicity. However, if the vein is not completely compressible then a thrombus is likely the cause, even if intravenous echogenic material cannot be seen.[2]

Doppler ultrasonography can be used to demonstrate decreased venous flow and a lack of response to distal vein augmentation (**Fig. 11**). Both findings may not locate the exact location of a thrombus, but do provide evidence that there is obstruction to venous flow between the compression point and the transducer.

Anatomy and Related Sonographic Findings for DVT

Understanding peripheral venous anatomy is required to perform an adequate sonographic examination for the diagnosis of DVT. Most DVTs will be found in the lower extremities, with only approximately 8% of all cases of DVT occurring in the upper

Table 1	
Wells criteria for the probability of DVT	
Clinical Features	**Score**
Active malignancy	1
Paralysis, paresis, lower extremity in cast	1
Bedridden ≥3 d or surgery in past 4 wk	1
Localized tenderness along deep veins	1
Entire leg swollen	1
Calf swollen >3 cm compared with opposite leg	1
Pitting edema greater in symptomatic leg	1
Superficial vein collaterals	1
Alternative diagnosis is more likely than DVT	−2

Table 2
Pretest probability of DVT and scores

Pretest Probability of DVT	Score
Low probability	<0
Moderate probability	1–2
High probability	>2

extremity.[4] Most upper extremity DVTs are associated with central lines, dialysis catheters, pacemakers, or clavicle fractures.[4] The veins with the greatest risk of causing pulmonary embolus (PE) are the common femoral vein (CFV), superficial femoral vein (SFV), and popliteal vein (PV). The SFV is part of the deep system (an unfortunate misnomer). The greater saphenous vein, on the other hand, is a superficial vein.

The PV is formed by a confluence of the anterior tibial vein (ATV), posterior tibial vein (PTV), and the peroneal vein in the lower leg. The PV passes through the adductor canal in the upper leg and becomes the SFV. This vessel joins the deep femoral vein (DFV) to form the CFV (**Fig. 12**). The DFV is not considered a source of PE, and therefore is not generally included in the sonographic evaluation for DVT. The CFV and SFV are medial to the femoral artery for approximately the first 5 cm distal to the inguinal ligament before tracking posterior to the artery as it makes its way toward the adductor canal. It is not uncommon to have duplication of the venous system in the lower extremity, particularly in the PVs.[5] Duplication of the PVs and SFVs is a normal variant previously reported in up to 25% of limbs.[5]

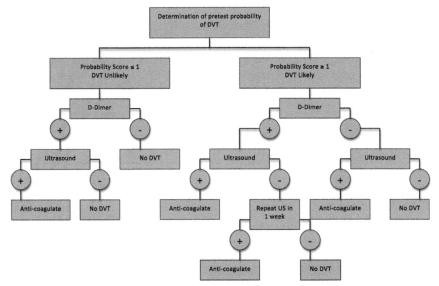

Fig. 8. Algorithm for the Wells criteria in combination with the D-dimer assay and ultrasonography for the evaluation of DVT.

> **Box 4**
> **Sonographic findings of DVT**
>
> Noncompressible vein
>
> Intraluminal echogenic material
>
> Decreased flow by Doppler ultrasonography
>
> Decreased distal augmentation

To perform the ultrasound examination, position the patient on a flat stretcher in the reverse Trendelenburg position so that the lower extremity is in a dependent position. Externally rotate the hip and flex the knee about 30° to allow access to the CFC, SFV, and PV (**Fig. 13**).

Sonographic evaluation of the lower extremity focuses on structures that present the greatest risk for DVT and subsequent PE. The veins distal to the PV are not consistently examined because calf vein thrombi are rare sources of clinically significant PE.[6,7] Ninety percent of all cases of acute PE are due to emboli emanating from the proximal rather than distal veins, veins or below the knee.[8] Up to 25% of distal DVTs may propagate into proximal veins, therefore increasing the risk for PE.[9] Current practice guidelines recommend that patients with a moderate to high pretest probability and a negative ultrasonography study should have a repeat sonogram in 5 to 7 days to assess for propagation of undetected distal DVT.[1,10]

In most vascular laboratories, a systematic examination of the entire extent of the CFV, SFC, and PV is performed on each leg. However, newer protocols used by clinicians (ie, nonradiologists or ultrasound technicians) examine only 2 or 3 areas of each leg using CUS without Doppler techniques. The areas examined include the CFV, the proximal SFV, and the PV. The clinicians performing the examinations are provided with a relatively small amount of training, yet their results compare favorably with those of the comprehensive ultrasound examinations performed by vascular laboratories.[11]

Approximately 8% of DVTs are located in the upper extremities.[4] The upper extremity has 3 large superficial veins: the antecubital, basilic, and cephalic. The deep veins of the arm are the brachial veins, which lie deep to the basilic vein. The brachial veins become

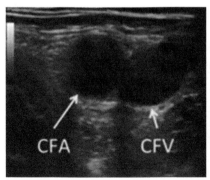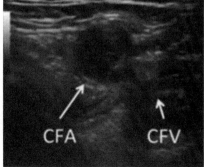

Fig. 9. Compression ultrasound (CUS) testing for DVT. The image on the left is the common femoral artery and vein. Gentle pressure causes complete apposition of the superficial and deep walls of the vein.

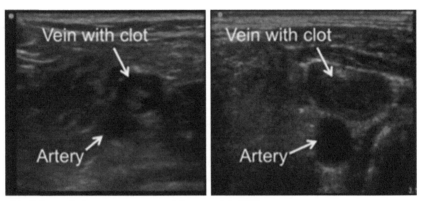

Fig. 10. Echogenic intravenous material seen with DVT.

the axillary veins as one moves proximally. The axillary veins coalesce and join the cephalic vein to become the subclavian vein (**Fig. 14**). The subclavian vein courses under the clavicle, making it challenging to compress in the evaluation for DVT.

The upper extremity is examined by ultrasonography with the patient in the supine position. The arm is abducted and externally rotated at the shoulder, and flexed at the elbow (**Fig. 15**). The examiner should scan from the antecubital fossa to the axilla and over the chest along the path of the subclavian vein. Although compression techniques are used, portions of the subclavian vein behind the clavicle cannot be compressed, and greater reliance on Doppler evaluation is required.[12]

With all duplicated venous systems of the upper and lower extremities, the examiner must make sure that both of the duplicated veins are examined for evidence of venous thromboembolism. Nearly all patients will have paired brachial veins (**Fig. 16**). Duplication of the axillary vein has been observed in 17.5% of cadaveric upper extremities.[13]

Peripheral Artery Aneurysms

Aneurysms are defined as an increase in normal artery diameter of 50% or greater. Peripheral vascular aneurysms are seen in medium-caliber and large-caliber vessels, most commonly in the popliteal artery (PA) and femoral artery (FA). The clinical

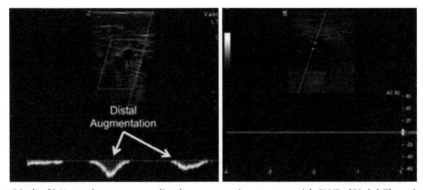

Fig. 11. (*Left*) Normal response to distal augmentation as seen with PWD. (*Right*) There is no venous flow and no response after compression of the vein distal to the location of the transducer.

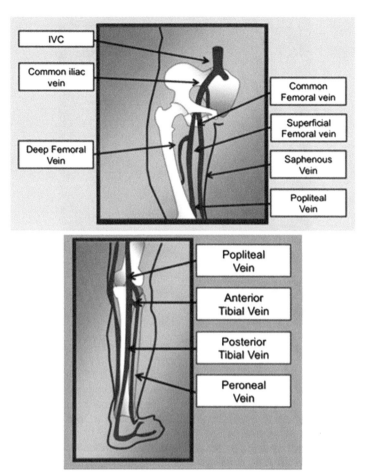

Fig. 12. Deep veins of the lower extremity. The common femoral vein (CFV) bifurcates into the superficial femoral vein (SFV) and deep femoral vein. The SFV becomes the popliteal vein (PV) once it emerges from the adductor canal. The PV trifurcates into the anterior tibial vein, posterior tibial vein, and peroneal vein. IVC, inferior vena cava.

presentation of peripheral artery aneurysms relates directly to arterial insufficiency caused by thrombosis, embolization, or rupture of the vessel, manifested by signs and symptoms ranging from claudication to limb ischemia.

PA aneurysms account for approximately 80% of all peripheral artery aneurysms. The PA is the distal continuation of the common FA (CFA), and ranges in size from 7 to 11 mm.[14] The popliteal artery lies deep to the PV, but may still be palpated in the popliteal fossa. This palpation is best done with the knee in a partially flexed position.

A bounding, easily palpated pulse in this region is suggestive of the presence of a PA aneurysm. When present, these aneurysms usually measure greater than 20 mm in diameter,[15] and their presentation usually includes limb ischemia and an easily palpable pulse. However, not all PA aneurysms are palpable, particularly if they are less than 20 mm in size or contain a thrombus. PA aneurysms larger than 20 mm have a higher risk of causing thromboembolic events. Unlike aortic aneurysms, the growth rate of PA aneurysms is difficult to predict.[16] PA aneurysms are found

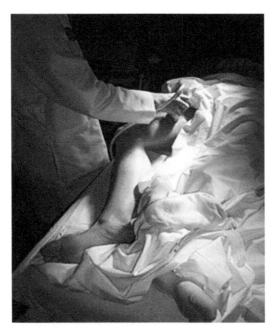

Fig. 13. Ultrasound examination technique for the lower extremity. The leg is externally rotated at the hip and the knee is flexed at approximately 30°, thus allowing access to the CFV, SFV, and PV.

bilaterally in approximately 50% of cases and are associated with abdominal aortic aneurysms approximately 40% of the time.[15] Therefore, patients diagnosed with PA aneurysms should undergo evaluation of the contralateral popliteal fossa, bilateral femoral arteries, and the aorta.[15]

Duplex ultrasonography is the preferred initial imaging modality for the evaluation of a PA aneurysm. This imaging is performed using both 2-dimensional and Doppler

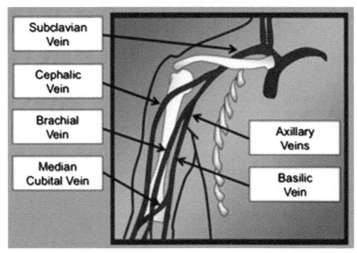

Fig. 14. The venous system of the upper extremity consists of several large veins in the upper arm: the cephalic vein, basilic vein, and brachial vein. The brachial vein is often duplicated.

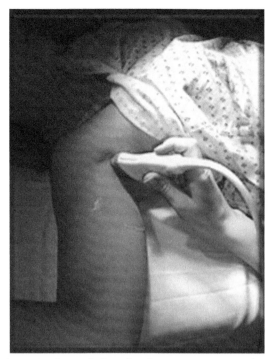

Fig. 15. Ultrasound examination technique for the upper extremity. The patient is in the supine position. The shoulder is abducted and externally rotated. The elbow is flexed.

sonography. B-mode is used for the measurement of vessel size to determine the presence of an aneurysm and whether a coexisting thrombus is present. Doppler ultrasonography is used to differentiate the PA from the PV, and to elucidate how much of the aneurysm is composed of atherosclerotic plaque or thrombus versus patent vascular lumen (**Fig. 17**).

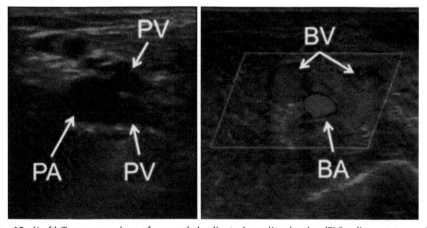

Fig. 16. (*Left*) Transverse view of normal duplicated popliteal veins (PV) adjacent to popliteal artery (PA). (*Right*) Transverse view of the brachial artery (BA) deep to duplicated brachial veins (BV), which have DVT.

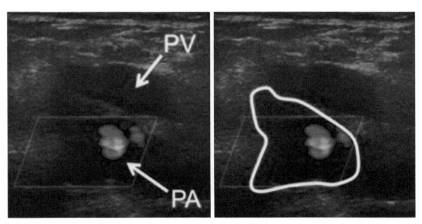

Fig. 17. (*Left*) Longitudinal view of the popliteal vein (PV) and artery (PA). The artery has an aneurysm. (*Right*) The same view with the aneurysm outlined in yellow. In this example a relatively small component of the aneurysm is patent lumen. The remainder of the PA aneurysm is atherosclerotic plaque and/or thrombus.

Doppler ultrasonography can also be used to differentiate aneurysm from nonvascular masses. Baker cysts are common nonvascular masses that may be seen during an evaluation for a potential PA aneurysm. This lesion is a nonvascular fluid collection, located in the popliteal fossa, which can be confused with a PA aneurysm. These cysts of the synovial bursa of the knee are usually created by knee disorders such as arthritis or cartilaginous injury (ie, meniscal tear). When they become inflamed or rupture, Baker cysts can cause a significant amount of pain and swelling. Using Duplex ultrasonography, the examiner can differentiate the arterial and venous popliteal vasculature from the cyst (**Figs. 18** and **19**). The cyst appears on the sonogram as an anechoic mass that may include echogenic debris or septations, but will not contain vascular flow.[17]

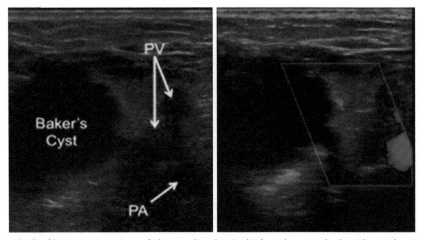

Fig. 18. (*Left*) Transverse view of the popliteal vein (PV) and artery (PA) with a Baker cyst. (*Right*) The same view with color flow over the artery and partially over the cyst. There is no flow present in the cyst.

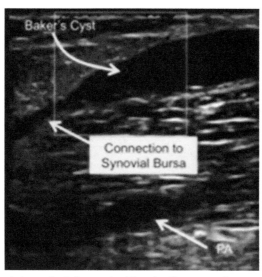

Fig. 19. Longitudinal view of a Baker cyst with color flow over the cyst cavity. Below this is the popliteal artery. The connection to the synovial bursa of the knee is seen at the far left of the cyst.

Pseudoaneurysms

Pseudoaneurysms are a result of vessel catheterization, trauma, infection, or disruption of an anastomosis (**Box 5**). Pseudoaneurysms involve a disruption in all 3 layers of the arterial wall and are contained by extravascular structures. Because they are not located within the arterial wall they are not true aneurysms, hence the name.

Pseudoaneurysms may occur in any location, but are most commonly encountered in the CFA following catheterization. The incidence of occurrence after catheterization is 0.5% to 2.0% after a diagnostic catheterization, which increases to 2.0% to 6.0% after an interventional procedure.[18] Interventional procedures are responsible for more than 80% of postcatheterization pseudoaneurysms.[19]

Pseudoaneurysms typically present as a pulsatile mass adjacent to an area of recent trauma, and must be differentiated from a hematoma or true aneurysm. Recent catheterization strongly favors pseudoaneurysm over true aneurysm. Medical management varies dramatically based on the diagnosis. Hematomas typically resolve spontaneously and require no further intervention. Pseudoaneurysms often require management by ultrasound-guided compression, ultrasound-guided thrombin injection, or surgical repair.

Box 5
Causes of pseudoaneurysm

After catheterization

Vessel wall rupture

Leaking surgical anastomosis

Direct trauma

Infection

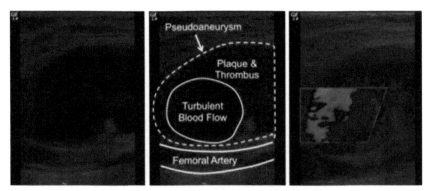

Fig. 20. Longitudinal view of pseudoaneurysm. There is a central area of turbulent blood flow seen by color flow.

Duplex ultrasonography is the standard for visualization of pseudoaneurysms. Typically the examiner will see a hematoma with variable echogenicity and turbulent pulsatile flow (**Fig. 20**).

It is important to scan very carefully through areas that are concerning for either a hematoma or a pseudoaneurysm, as the 2 structures can appear remarkably similar on ultrasonography. To confirm the presence of a pseudoaneurysm, direct visualization of the connection between the extravascular collection of blood and the artery is required. PWD should be used to confirm flow into the pseudoaneurysm during systole, and out of the pseudoaneurysm during diastole.[20]

Arterial Occlusion of Extremities

Acute limb ischemia is defined as a decrease in limb perfusion that results in jeopardized limb viability. Despite improvements in management, limb ischemia continues to cause significant morbidity and mortality. Revascularization of an ischemic limb within 12 hours still has an amputation rate of 6%. At 24 hours, the amputation rate increases to 20%.

Limb ischemia typically results from embolus, thrombus, or trauma (**Boxes 6** and **7, Table 3**). Emboli are most commonly found in an area with arterial narrowing or an arterial branch point. Less common causes of limb ischemia include external compression of the artery (compartment syndrome, vascular dissection), vasospasm, and vasculitis.

Ischemia should be considered in those presenting with pain at rest, ulcers, or gangrene. Pain usually begins distally in the extremity and progresses proximally as

---

Box 6
Thrombotic causes of acute arterial occlusion of an extremity

Vascular grafts

Atherosclerosis

Thrombosis of aneurysm

Entrapment syndrome

Hypercoagulable state

Low flow rate

Box 7
Traumatic causes of acute arterial occlusion of an extremity

Blunt trauma

Penetrating trauma

Iatrogenic (needle cannulation)

---

the ischemia increases. The pain may subside later in the presentation, secondary to progressive ischemic nerve damage and sensory loss.

The skin should be examined for the presence of pallor, temperature, and capillary refill. If pallor is present, a line of demarcation should be identified. Signs of chronic ischemia such as hair loss, skin atrophy, and thickened nails should also be noted. A detailed neurologic examination of the extremity should be performed to assess motor and sensory function. Sensory deficits to the dorsum of the foot are often the first identified.

Evaluation of pulses should begin with the contralateral side to establish a baseline. A normal contralateral pulse suggests no preexisting arterial disease. In this situation, embolism is the most likely cause of ischemia. A decreased pulse in the contralateral extremity suggests preexisting peripheral vascular disease and chronic limb ischemia. In this situation, thrombosis is the more likely source of the ischemia (**Box 8**).

In patients with normal pulses, other causes should also be considered. Radiculopathy from spinal stenosis can produce pseudoclaudication, and symptoms can be induced by walking and relieved by rest and leaning forward. Acute disk herniation can also result in lower extremity pain secondary to nerve-root impingement. Phlegmasia cerulea dolens is an uncommon, severe form of DVT, causing pain, edema, and cyanosis to the extremity.

Ultrasonography of the extremity's arterial supply is a noninvasive technique that provides valuable information obtained in real time at the bedside. A detailed ultrasound examination of a lower extremity for occlusion and stenosis is time consuming and can take more than 30 minutes when performed by an experienced sonographer. A focused examination evaluating only for evidence of arterial occlusion in the lower extremity can be performed quickly at the bedside.[21] However, ultrasonography performed by Emergency or Critical Care physicians for acute arterial occlusion has not yet been extensively studied.

Sonographic evaluation of the arterial system in the setting of possible limb ischemia is performed using a high-frequency linear-array transducer. Both 2-dimensional and Doppler ultrasonography are used to identify the vessel, evaluate the vessel wall, document blood flow, and look for thrombus (**Fig. 21**).

Table 3
Embolic causes of acute arterial occlusion of an extremity

Cardiac Source	Arterial Source	Paradoxic Embolus
Atrial fibrillation	Aneurysm	Patent foramen ovale
Myocardial infarction	Atherosclerotic plaque	Atrial septal defect
Endocarditis	Dissection	Ventricular septal defect
Valvular disease		
Atrial myxoma		
Prosthetic valves		

Box 8
The 6 Ps of limb ischemia
Pain
Pallor
Pulselessness
Paralysis
Paresthesias
Poikilothermia

PWD is used to describe blood flow in terms of flow rate, vessel stenosis, and obstruction. Normal flow rates for lower extremity arteries are listed in **Table 4**.[22]

Normal arterial blood flow with PWD is described as triphasic (**Figs. 22–24**).

With arterial stenosis, the blood flow at the stenotic segment increases with loss of the normal triphasic appearance on PWD. Distal to the stenosis the flow rates are decreased and the flow pattern appears monophasic, with decreasing levels of blood flow from stenosis and obstruction.

With higher flow rates, aliasing may appear. Aliasing occurs when velocities exceed the Doppler measured limit, and appears as reverse color flow. Visualization of the vessel distant to the stenotic area will display a mosaic pattern, representing turbulent flow. On PWD the waveform will exceed the measured limit, and appear at the opposite side of the spectral analysis.

For the ultrasound examination of the lower extremity arterial system (**Fig. 25**), the patient is placed in the same position as for the evaluation of DVT. The CFA begins at the inguinal ligament and is lateral to the CFV. The CFA proceeds in a linear course adjacent to the CFV. The first branch point of the femoral artery is the deep femoral artery. After this bifurcation the vessel continues as the superficial femoral artery (SFA), anterior to the SFV. At the adductor canal, the SFA and SFV track posteriorly and become the PA and PV.

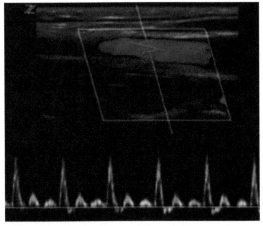

Fig. 21. Duplex imaging with PWD demonstrating a normal artery contour and normal triphasic arterial waveform.

Table 4
Normal peripheral arterial peak systolic velocities

Common femoral	90–120 cm/s
Superficial femoral	75–100 cm/s
Popliteal	60–80 cm/s
Tibial	30–70 cm/s

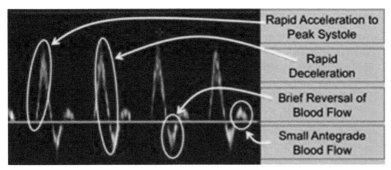

Fig. 22. Normal triphasic arterial waveform with PWD.

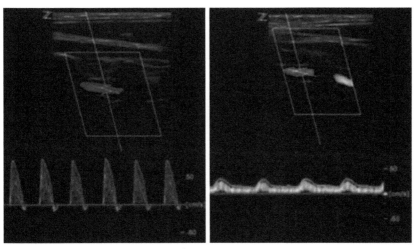

Fig. 23. (*Left*) The sampling volume is located at an arterial stenosis. PWD indicates a higher velocity than expected and a loss of the normal triphasic waveform. (*Right*) A very low rate of arterial blood flow is seen. The PWD indicates low velocity with a monophasic blood flow waveform. This area is distal to an arterial stenosis.

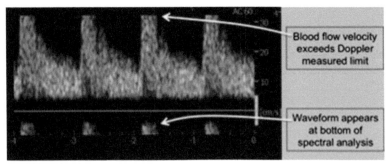

Fig. 24. When blood flow velocity exceeds the Doppler measured limit, the waveform aliases and appears on the opposite side of the spectral analysis.

The PA travels behind the knee and is deep to the PV. The PA divides into the anterior and posterior tibial arteries below the knee. The posterior tibial artery (PTA) is evaluated in same position as used for imaging of the PA. The PTA courses along the posteromedial aspect of the lower leg and lies just medial to the fibula. The anterior tibial artery is evaluated with the patient in the supine position. The vessel is at the

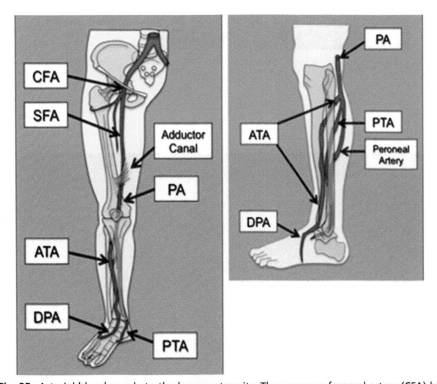

Fig. 25. Arterial blood supply to the lower extremity. The common femoral artery (CFA) bifurcates into the superficial femoral artery (SFA) and deep femoral artery. The SFA passes through the adductor canal and emerges behind the knee as the popliteal artery (PA). The PA trifurcates into the posterior tibial artery (PTA), anterior tibial artery (ATA), and peroneal artery. DPA, dorsalis pedis artery.

anterolateral portion of the lower leg, and becomes the dorsalis pedis artery (DPA) on the dorsal surface of the foot.

The examiner should look for evidence of abnormal blood flow at several key locations including the CFA, SFA (at its origin, middle, and distal segment), PA, DPA, and distal PTA at the medial malleolus.

SUMMARY

Venous thromboembolic disease is one of the most prevalent medical problems plaguing emergency and critical care patients. Physicians who enhance their clinical skills with bedside ultrasonography not only improve and expedite the care of seriously ill patients but also reduce the considerable morbidity and mortality associated with DVT and PE. The key pieces of knowledge include using pretest probability, being familiar with the peripheral venous anatomy, and knowledge of the procedures involved with scanning extremities for potential thrombus.

Although peripheral aneurysm, pseudoaneurysm, and acute arterial occlusion are not nearly as prevalent as DVT, the associated complications are just as great. Having the ability to quickly assess the patient at the bedside has the potential to significantly reduce the time to treatment and helps in notifying the appropriate consultant. Knowing how to perform arterial ultrasonography to evaluate for limb and life-threatening conditions can improve patient care and outcomes.

REFERENCES

1. Wells PS, Anderson DR, Bormanis J, et al. Value of assessment of pretest probability of deep vein thrombosis in clinical management. Lancet 1997;350:1795–8.
2. Heijboer H, Jongbloets LM, Buller HR, et al. Clinical utility of real-time compression ultrasonography for diagnostic management of patients with recurrent venous thrombosis. Acta Radiol 1992;33:297–300.
3. Frazee B, Snoey E, Levitt A. Emergency department compression ultrasound to diagnose proximal deep vein thrombosis. J Emerg Med 2001;20(2):107–12.
4. Greben C, Charles H. Imaging in Deep Venous Thrombosis of the Upper Extremity. eMedicine. Available at: http://emedicine.medscape.com/article/421151. Accessed November 2013.
5. Dona E, Fletcher JP, Hughes TM, et al. Duplicated popliteal and superficial femoral veins: incidence and potential significance. ANZ J Surg 2000;70(6):438–40.
6. Kakkar W, Howes J, Sharma V, et al. A comparative double-blind randomised trial of a new second generation LMWH (bemiparin). J Thromb Haemost 2000;83(4):523–9.
7. Kearon C. Initial treatment of venous thromboembolism. J Thromb Haemost 1999;82(2):887–91.
8. Galanaud JP, Sevestre-Pietri MA, Bosson JL, et al. Comparative study on risk factors and early outcome of symptomatic distal versus proximal deep vein thrombosis: results from the OPTIMEV study. J Thromb Haemost 2009;102:493.
9. Lagersted CI, Olsson CG, Fagher BO, et al. Need for long-term anticoagulation treatment in symptomatic calf-vein thrombosis. Lancet 1985;2(8454):515–8.
10. Wells PS, Anderson DR, Rodger M, et al. Evaluation of D-dimer in the diagnosis of suspected deep vein thrombosis. N Engl J Med 2003;349(13):1227–35.
11. Crisp JG, Lovato LM, Jang TB. Compression Ultrasonography of the lower extremity with portable vascular ultrasonography can accurately detect deep venous thrombosis in the emergency department. Ann Emerg Med 2010;56(6):601–10.

12. Tapson VF, Carroll BA, Davidson BL, et al. The diagnostic approach to acute venous thromboembolism. Official statement of the American Thoracic Society. Am J Respir Crit Care Med 1999;160(3):1043–66.
13. Yang HJ, Gil YC, Jin JD, et al. Novel findings of anatomy and variations of the axillary vein and its tributaries. Clin Anat 2012;25(7):893–902.
14. Wolf YG, Kobzantsev Z, Zelmanovich L. Size of normal and aneurysmal popliteal arteries: a duplex ultrasound study. J Vasc Surg 2006;43(3):488–92.
15. Thompson MM, Bell PF. ABC of arterial and venous disease: arterial aneurysms. BMJ 2000;320:1193–6.
16. Magee R, Quigley F, McCann M, et al. Growth and the risk factors for expansion of dilated popliteal arteries. Eur J Vasc Endovasc Surg 2010;39(5):606–11.
17. Torreggiani WC, Al-Ismail K, Munk PL, et al. The imaging spectrum of Baker's (popliteal) cysts. Clin Radiol 2002;57:681.
18. Hessel SJ, Adams DF, Abrams HL. Complications of angiography. Radiology 1981;138:273–81.
19. Webber GW, Jang J, Gustavson S, et al. Contemporary management of postcatheterization pseudoaneurysms. Circulation 2007;115:2666–74.
20. Rozen G, Samuels DR, Blank A. The to and fro sign: the hallmark of pseudoaneurysm. Isr Med Assoc J 2001;3:781–2.
21. Watanabe R, Nakanishi K, Ochi S, et al. Assessment of lower limb artery disease by ultrasound imaging. Rinsho Byori 2007;55(2):159–69.
22. Reynolds T, editor. The echocardiographer's pocket reference. Phoenix (AZ): Arizona Heart Institute; 2007.

Bedside Ultrasonography for Obstetric and Gynecologic Emergencies

Aparajita Sohoni, MD*, Justin Bosley, MD, Jacob C. Miss, MD

KEYWORDS

- Ultrasonography • Obstetric • Gynecologic • Emergency imaging
- Ectopic pregnancy • Yolk sac • Gestational sac

KEY POINTS

- This article reviews the basic technique of performing transabdominal and transvaginal (endocavitary) ultrasonography.
- The sonographic appearance of a normal intrauterine pregnancy, as well as abnormal findings that may be encountered, are reviewed.
- A range of common ovarian and uterine diseases are reviewed.

INTRODUCTION

Ultrasonography is the ideal diagnostic modality for evaluation of a female patient with a pelvic complaint.[1] This article of *Critical Care Clinics* provides a guide for using bedside ultrasonography for the diagnosis of emergent obstetric and gynecologic disease. First, how to perform the scans is reviewed. This review is followed by a detailed discussion of the appearance of a normal intrauterine pregnancy (IUP) versus an abnormal one, including reviews of fetal bradycardia, ectopic pregnancies, and molar pregnancy. Subsequently, common gynecologic complaints, including ovarian cysts, uterine fibroids, and intrauterine device (IUD) localization, are reviewed. Emergent gynecologic diseases, including ovarian torsion, tubo-ovarian abscess (TOA), hydrosalpinx, and pyosalpinx, are discussed. Readers should gain from this article an understanding of how to perform these scans and should be able to apply this knowledge to the clinical scenarios they encounter.

Disclosure: The authors have identified no disclosures in terms of funding sources or conflicts of interest for themselves or their spouse/partner.
Department of Emergency Medicine, Highland Hospital, Alameda County Medical Center, 1411 East 31st Street, Oakland, CA 94602, USA
* Corresponding author.
E-mail address: sohoni79@gmail.com

Crit Care Clin 30 (2014) 207–226
http://dx.doi.org/10.1016/j.ccc.2013.10.002   **criticalcare.theclinics.com**
0749-0704/14/$ – see front matter © 2014 Elsevier Inc. All rights reserved.

TECHNICAL CONSIDERATIONS OF OBSTETRIC AND GYNECOLOGIC SONOGRAPHY
Transducer Selection

Ultrasonographic images of the female pelvis can be obtained using either a curvilinear or an endocavitary transducer (**Fig. 1**).

The decision of which transducer to use should be based on the clinical scenario and the diagnostic question the provider seeks to answer, along with the comfort of the provider with performing either scan. For example, in a pregnant patient in the first trimester for whom the provider seeks to document the presence or absence of an IUP, an endocavitary approach provides the most information as well as the most detailed view of the structures of interest. In a 50-year-old woman with vaginal bleeding, a transabdominal view using the curvilinear transducer is likely sufficient to evaluate for the presence of obvious causes of her dysfunctional uterine bleeding. In general, the endocavitary transducer should be used for performing ultrasonography in the first trimester of pregnancy and for evaluation of ovarian or fallopian tube disease.[2–4] The low-frequency, curvilinear transducer can be used for evaluation of second-trimester or third-trimester fetuses, and larger uterine and ovarian diseases, such as fibroids, large ovarian cysts, and so forth.[5] However, these are generalizations, and physician comfort with the scan is an obvious key factor in determining which scan to perform in which clinical context.[6] The next section reviews the steps of performing each scan.

TECHNIQUE FOR PERFORMING TRANSABDOMINAL PELVIC ULTRASONOGRAPHY

Transabdominal pelvic ultrasonography should be performed with the patient in the supine position. The curvilinear 3-MHz to 5-MHz transducer should be placed in a transverse orientation just proximal to the symphysis pubis, with the transducer indicator toward the patient's right side. Begin by identifying the full bladder, and then note the outline of the uterine wall and the endometrial stripe immediately posterior to the bladder (**Fig. 2**).

Note that the absence of a full bladder significantly limits the examination, because the anechoic urine filling the bladder is serving as the acoustic window to allow better visualization of the deeper-lying uterus. Fan the transducer superiorly to inferiorly, and evaluate, or interrogate, the uterus for any pertinent findings. Repeat the examination with the transducer indicator pointing toward the patient's head, in the sagittal

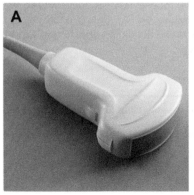
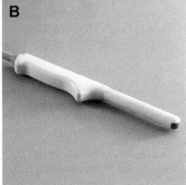

Fig. 1. (*A*) Curvilinear (2–5 MHz) and (*B*) endocavitary (5–8 MHz) transducers. (*Courtesy of* FUJIFILM Sonosite, San Francisco, CA; with permission.)

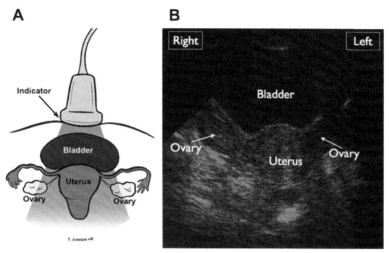

Fig. 2. Transabdominal pelvic ultrasonography shown in the transverse plane with the probe indicator pointing toward the patient's right side. (*A*) Schematic and (*B*) ultrasonographic image showing labeled structures. (*Courtesy of* Sonia Johnson, MD, Los Angeles, CA and FUJIFILM Sonosite, San Francisco, CA.)

orientation, and fan the transducer from the patient's right side to the patient's left side (**Fig. 3**).

Again, interrogate the pelvic structures. Note that it is possible to evaluate the ovaries on transabdominal ultrasonography, if the patient has a full urinary bladder. It is easier to visualize the ovaries in thinner patients, or if there is significant disease, such as a large ovarian cyst. However, most providers find evaluating the ovaries easier on endocavitary ultrasonography.[7] However, if desired, evaluate each adnexa by maintaining the transducer in the transverse orientation, but angling the beams to the patient's right adnexa and fanning the transducer superiorly and inferiorly.

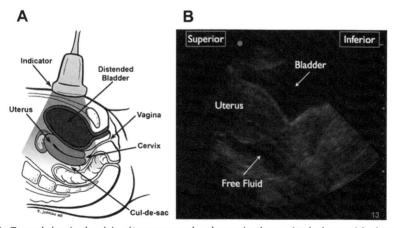

Fig. 3. Transabdominal pelvic ultrasonography shown in the sagittal plane with the probe indicator pointing toward the patient's head. (*A*) Schematic and (*B*) ultrasonographic image showing labeled structures. (*Courtesy of* Sonia Johnson, MD, Los Angeles, CA and FUJIFILM Sonosite, San Francisco, CA.)

Repeat the same procedure with the beams angling toward the patient's left adnexa (**Fig. 4**).

TECHNIQUE FOR PERFORMING ENDOCAVITARY PELVIC ULTRASONOGRAPHY

Endocavitary pelvic ultrasonography should be performed with the patient in the lithotomy position. It is imperative that the patient empties her bladder before endocavitary ultrasonography is performed, both for patient comfort and for better sonographic visualization of the target structures. During endocavitary ultrasonography, the bladder is not being used as a sonographic or acoustic window. In this examination, the goal is to place the endocavitary transducer directly against the structures being interrogated (ie, uterus and ovaries). A full bladder displaces the uterus posteriorly, making access to the uterus by the endocavitary transducer difficult. An empty bladder enables the uterus to move anteriorly and superiorly, where it can be easily interrogated by the endocavitary transducer. For this reason, most providers perform transabdominal ultrasonography first, when the patient's bladder is full, and then have the patient empty her bladder before endocavitary ultrasonography is performed.

The endocavitary transducer should be introduced with the transducer indicator pointing toward the ceiling. Insert the transducer into the patient's vagina and move toward the cervix. The depth of insertion is unique to each patient, and therefore, it is imperative to monitor the ultrasound screen as the probe is being inserted. Look for the bladder superiorly, the uterus in the center of the screen, and the cervix to the right of the screen (**Fig. 5**).

With the probe indicator pointing anteriorly toward the patient's pubic symphysis, you see a sagittal view of the pelvis. Find the endometrial stripe running through the uterus, and use that location as the midpoint of the scan. From this position, with the endometrial stripe in sagittal view, fan the transducer from the patient's right to the patient's left, and note any abnormal findings.

After completing the sagittal views of the pelvis, rotate the transducer 90° counterclockwise, so that the indicator is pointing toward the patient's right side. This rotation provides a transverse, or coronal, view of the pelvis. Again, position the transducer so that the uterus is midline and the endometrial stripe runs from left to right along the center of the screen. Then, fan the transducer anteriorly and posteriorly, moving smoothly through the uterus in a transverse fashion (**Fig. 6**).

To evaluate the adnexa, maintain a coronal orientation and angle the transducer to the patient's right adnexa. Fan the transducer anteriorly and posteriorly, and note the

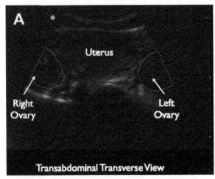
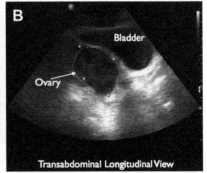

Fig. 4. Transabdominal imaging of ovaries. (*A*) Probe indicator toward patient's right side and (*B*) probe indicator toward patient's head.

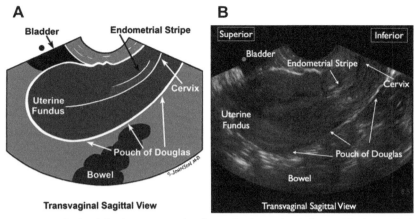

Fig. 5. Transvaginal pelvic ultrasonography shown in the sagittal plane with the probe indicator toward the ceiling. (*A*) Schematic and (*B*) ultrasonographic image showing labeled structures. (*Courtesy of* Sonia Johnson, MD, Los Angeles, CA.)

characteristic ovoid appearance of the ovary with areas of hypoechogenicity. This is the classic chocolate-chip cookie appearance of the ovary. It is often useful to find the broad ligament coming off the uterus and follow this structure laterally until you see the ovary. Repeat this scan of the left adnexa, using the same technique. Adding color flow to the image can be helpful in distinguishing the ovary from the adjacent uterine vessels. The color flow pattern of a normal ovary is distinct from the pulsatile or constant flow seen in uterine vessels (**Fig. 7**).

EMERGENCY ULTRASONOGRAPHY IN THE OBSTETRIC PATIENT

If a pregnant patient is being evaluated in the acute care setting, bedside ultrasonography focuses primarily on detecting an IUP and ruling out an ectopic pregnancy, followed by dating the fetus and characterizing its viability.[8,9] Additional diagnoses, such

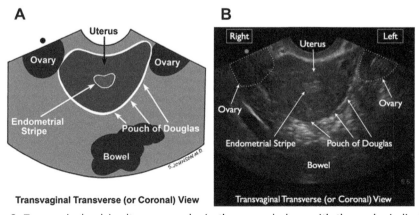

Fig. 6. Transvaginal pelvic ultrasonography in the coronal plane with the probe indicator pointing toward the patient's pubis symphysis. (*A*) Schematic and (*B*) ultrasonographic image showing labeled structures. (*Courtesy of* Sonia Johnson, MD, Los Angeles, CA.)

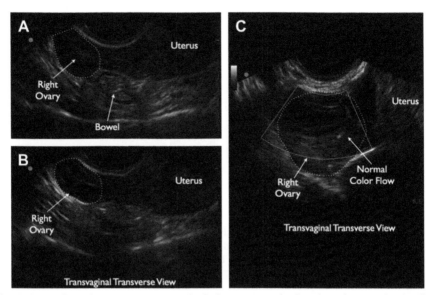

Fig. 7. Normal ovaries seen on transvaginal ultrasonography (*A*, *B*), with normal color flow pattern (*C*).

as molar pregnancies, the localization of an IUD in a pregnant patient, or the presence of multiple fetuses, can also be made easily at the bedside.[10–14]

DETECTING A NORMAL IUP

When following the steps below, providers must first ensure that the structure they are visualizing (eg, the double decidual sac sign [DDSS], gestational sac, yolk sac, fetal pole) is intrauterine and not extrauterine. Providers should first identify the uterine wall and ensure that the structure that they are interrogating lies within the borders of the uterus.

The first sonographic sign of pregnancy is the DDSS.[15,16] This sac is identifiable via endocavitary ultrasonography as early as 4 weeks and 3 days of gestation. The DDSS consists of 2 hyperechoic concentric rings surrounding an inner anechoic or hypoechoic gestational sac (**Fig. 8**). The outer layer is the decidua parietalis and the inner layer is the decidua capsularis.[15] At the earliest detection via ultrasonography, the DDSS diameter is usually 2 to 3 mm and increases by approximately 1.2 mm/d. Note that the presence of a DDSS does not represent an IUP. The presence of a yolk sac is the earliest finding of an IUP. The yolk sac, a single-walled small circular structure, forms within the gestational sac and should be present by the time the mean diameter of the DDSS measures 8 mm, or approximately 5 weeks of gestation (**Fig. 9**).

The mean diameter of the gestational sac is measured by taking 3 orthogonal measurements across the anechoic space of the gestational sac. A hyperechoic fetal pole should be seen at approximately 6 weeks of gestation or when the mean gestational sac diameter is greater than or equal to 16 mm (**Fig. 10**).

It is important that novice sonographers do not mistake a pseudogestational sac for a true gestational sac or DDSS. A pseudogestational sac is an anechoic sac with a thin ring that usually represents a small intrauterine fluid collection (**Fig. 11**). These pseudogestational sacs can be seen with an ectopic pregnancy. A pseudogestational sac

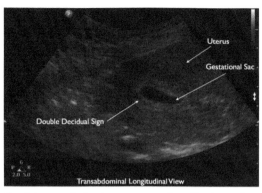

Fig. 8. DDSS: note the 2 hyperechoic rings surrounding the inner hypoechoic gestational sac, all located within the uterus.

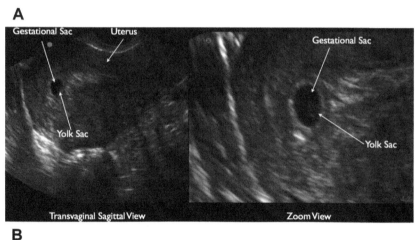

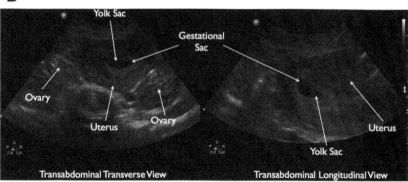

Fig. 9. (*A*) Yolk sac as seen on transvaginal ultrasonography with zoomed-in view provided. (*B*) Yolk sac as seen on transabdominal ultrasonography in transverse and longitudinal views.

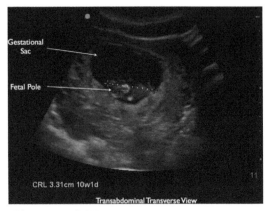

Fig. 10. Fetal pole with measured CRL.

does not have the characteristic DDSS, is usually located centrally within the uterus, and does not contain a yolk sac.[17]

CORRELATION WITH SERUM β-HUMAN CHORIONIC GONADOTROPIN LEVELS

The serum β-human chorionic gonadotropin (β-HCG) level can serve as a rough guide to which findings should be expected on endocavitary or transabdominal ultrasonography. **Table 1** correlates the serum levels with ultrasonographic findings and weeks of gestation, acknowledging that significant overlap exists between HCG ranges. If HCG levels are higher than expected for weeks of gestation, or do not correlate with sonographic findings, consider an ectopic pregnancy, multiple gestations, or a molar pregnancy.

FETAL DATING AND VIABILITY BY TRIMESTER

After confirming the presence of an IUP, it is important to date the fetus and assess for fetal viability. There are numerous methods to date the fetus, with the preferred method in the first trimester being the crown-rump length (CRL). In the second and third trimesters, the easiest measurements are the biparietal diameter (BPD) and

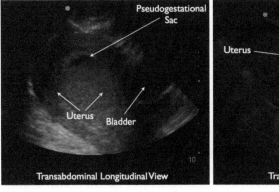
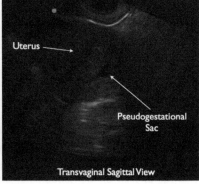

Fig. 11. Examples of pseudogestational sacs.

Table 1
Correlation of predicted HCG levels and expected sonographic findings with gestational age (GA) and mean gestational sac diameter (GSD)

GA (d)	Mean GSD (mm)	Predicted HCG Level (mIU/mL) (95% Confidence Interval)	Ultrasonographic Modality	Expected Sonographic Findings
31 (30–33)	5	1932 (1026–3636)	Endocavitary	Gestational sac
36 (34–38)	9	3785 (2085–6870)	Endocavitary	Yolk sac
41 (39–43)	15	10,379 (5766–18,682)	Endocavitary	Fetal pole and heart beat
49	19	20,337 (10,951–37,761)	Endocavitary, transabdominal	Embryonic torso and head

Data from Refs.[8,14,18]

femur length (FL). In addition, the tibia length (TL) can be measured, although for novice sonographers, the tibia is more difficult to isolate for measurement. Abdominal circumference is also a valid way to date the fetus but is more challenging for a novice sonographer to perform. **Table 2** reviews these techniques for fetal dating and shows the correlation of emergency medicine providers (EMP) performing fetal dating with fetal dating performed by senior obstetricians or obstetric ultrasonography technicians.

Fetal viability is determined by the presence of cardiac activity. Cardiac activity is first detectable at 5 to 6 weeks' gestation and when the CRL on endocavitary ultrasonography is greater than 5 mm. Fetal movement should be detected at this time in a normal fetus. Further prognostic information about the fetus can be gained by specifically measuring the heart rate. Fetal bradycardia increases the chance of miscarriage.

Table 2
Techniques to date a fetus by trimester

Trimester	Techniques to Date the Fetus (EMP Correlation[a])	Technique Detail
First	CRL (0.935)	CRL: place ultrasound calipers from the top of the head to the best-estimated region of the rump. Do not include the yolk sac or limbs
Second	BPD (0.947) FL (0.957) TL (N/A)	BPD: measure in a transverse (axial) plane at the level of the falx cerebri and the thalamus, placing calipers at the outer aspect of the skull in the near field and inner table of the skull in the far field
		FL: measure the full femoral diaphysis from 1 end to the other, disregarding any curvature, without including the distal epiphysis
		TL: measure the full diaphyseal length, avoid including the talocalcaneal complex
Third	FL (0.957) TL (N/A)	See above

Abbreviation: N/A, not applicable.
 [a] EMP correlation: EMPs performing fetal dating correlated with fetal dating performed by senior obstetricians or obstetric ultrasonography technicians.
 Data from Refs.[19–23]

The heart rates that signify bradycardia (represented by fetal heart rate [FHR] seen 2 standard deviations < the expected FHR for CRL length) vary with CRL measurements and are shown in **Table 3**. This information, although not necessarily critical to the management of the patient in the acute care setting, is of great value to the patient and to the patient's obstetrician during subsequent evaluations and follow-up.

If no heartbeat is seen, and the CRL is greater than 5 mm, the patient should be counseled that embryonic demise has occurred. This finding triggers a different sequence of events based on the gestational age. Obstetrics should be consulted to determine the correct course, because options include observation and expectant management, dilation and curettage, or medical therapy.

ECTOPIC PREGNANCY

If no IUP is visualized on endocavitary ultrasonography, the provider must evaluate for a possible ectopic pregnancy. Ectopic pregnancies are estimated to occur in 1% to 2% of pregnancies, but contribute to 3% to 4% of pregnancy-related mortality.[24,25] The cause is complex, but the most commonly recognized risk factors for ectopic pregnancy are previous ectopic pregnancy, acute or chronic pelvic inflammatory disease, previous tubal surgery, and hormonal manipulations.[26] Ectopic pregnancies most frequently implant in the fallopian tube, with implantation in the interstitial portion of the fallopian tube, abdominal cavity, ovary, or cesarean scar comprising less than 10% of cases.[27] Most patients with an ectopic pregnancy present before rupture, and generally have nonspecific complaints similar to those seen with viable IUP or miscarriage (eg, first-trimester bleeding, abdominal/pelvic pain).[27,28]

From a sonographic standpoint, the provider should consider whether the patient clinically appears to have a ruptured or unruptured ectopic pregnancy. A ruptured ectopic pregnancy can result in considerable intraperitoneal exsanguination, hypotension, tachycardia, and abdominal pain. The patient likely appears uncomfortable and critically ill. In the critically ill patient, bedside ultrasonography should begin with a scan of the abdomen and pelvis to evaluate for any intraperitoneal free fluid. Start with a low-frequency, curvilinear, or phased array transducer and scan the right upper quadrant (Morrison pouch) and pouch of Douglas (**Fig. 12**).

The detection of free fluid in the abdomen of a pregnant patient who appears ill should trigger immediate obstetric consultation for a likely ruptured ectopic pregnancy, because 1 study showed an increased likelihood ratio of 112 for operative intervention in patients with a ruptured ectopic pregnancy who had free fluid in that location.[29] Although other causes, such as a ruptured hemorrhagic cyst in the setting of a normal IUP, can also cause this presentation, this is less likely, and the novice

Table 3		
FHR correlated with CRL		
50th Percentile CRL (mm)	**Range of Expected 50th Percentile FHR**	**<5% Expected FHR**
<5	100–120	<100
5–9	120–140	100–120
10–15	140–160	120–140

Data from Papaioannou GI, Syngelaki A, Poon LC, et al. Normal ranges of embryonic length, embryonic heart rate, gestational sac diameter and yolk sac diameter at 6–10 weeks. Fetal Diagn Ther 2010;28(4):212–4; and Varelas FK, Prapas NM, Liang RI, et al. Yolk sac size and embryonic heart rate as prognostic factors of first trimester pregnancy outcome. Eur J Obstet Gynecol Reprod Biol 2008;138(1):11.

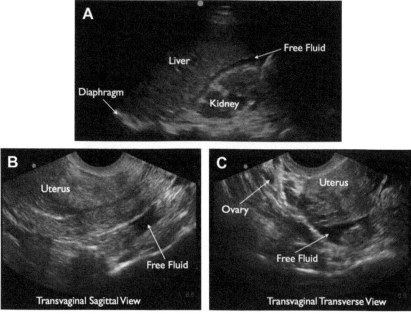

Fig. 12. Free fluid in Morrison pouch (A) and pouch of Douglas (B, C).

sonographer should not delay consultation to parse this out. If the sonographer is experienced, and the patient is stable despite the presence of free fluid in the Morrison pouch, investigation of the uterus using the same transabdominal transducer can confirm the absence of an IUP, or, if there is an IUP, suggest a ruptured hemorrhagic cyst or the rare heterotopic pregnancy. Regardless, a prompt and urgent obstetric consultation should be made.

Unruptured ectopic pregnancies pose a diagnostic challenge in the acute care setting. These patients present with vague symptoms such as pain in the lower abdomen or adnexa, and often have β-HCG levels that are in the discriminatory zone. In these patients, a thorough scan of the adnexa using the endocavitary transducer may show an adnexal mass that represents an unruptured ectopic pregnancy. In addition, careful evaluation of the uterus and cervix may show findings such as a pseudogestational sac, which suggests an ectopic pregnancy, or visualization of an ectopic pregnancy implanted at the cervix or other abnormal location (**Fig. 13**).

If an ectopic pregnancy is visualized, the obstetrics team should be consulted for appropriate management. If the patient has abdominal or pelvic pain, and a positive pregnancy test, and neither an IUP nor ectopic pregnancy can be visualized on ultrasonography, the provider should follow institution-specific guidelines to monitor the patient. The patient should be counseled that she has an indeterminate study and is at risk for having an ectopic pregnancy. In most clinical situations, repeat ultrasonography and repeat HCG level should be obtained within 48 hours, and the patient should be provided with specific return and follow-up instructions. Most providers do not feel comfortable with bedside ultrasonography alone in this clinical scenario. Typically, these patients warrant comprehensive ultrasonography performed by radiology with ultrasound machines that have better imaging capabilities.

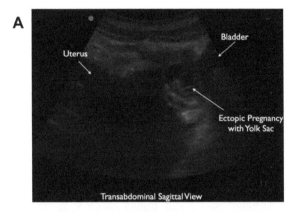

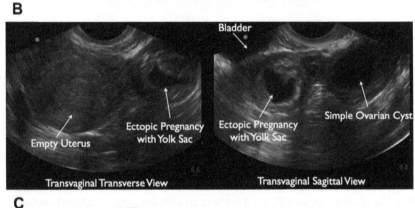

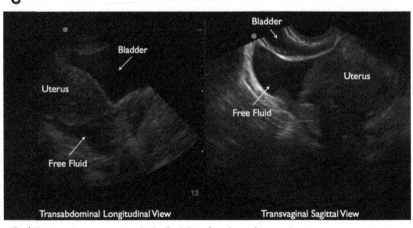

Fig. 13. (*A*) Ectopic pregnancy (tubal). (*B*) Left adnexal ectopic as seen on transverse and sagittal views, with adjacent ovary and ovarian cyst. (*C*) Ruptured ectopic pregnancy showing free fluid in the pelvis.

HETEROTOPIC PREGNANCY

Given the rare incidence of heterotopic pregnancies (1 in 30,000 pregnancies), the visualization of an IUP normally halts the search for an ectopic pregnancy.[30]

Obviously, this situation does not apply to patients who have undergone assisted reproduction techniques, such as hormone-induced superovulation, intrauterine insemination, or in vitro fertilization. In these populations, the reported incidence of heterotopic pregnancy is 1 in 3900 pregnancies.[31–33] Providers performing pelvic ultrasonography on these patients should be aware of the increased incidence of heterotopic pregnancies and should carefully interrogate the adnexa for any masses that may represent a heterotopic pregnancy in symptomatic patients.

GESTATIONAL TROPHOBLASTIC DISEASE

Gestational trophoblastic disease (GTD) includes the diagnoses of complete or partial hydatidiform moles, gestational trophoblastic neoplasia, choriocarcinoma, and placental site trophoblastic tumors. Complete and partial hydatidiform moles comprise 90% of cases of GTD. The feared complication, aside from failing to diagnosis these conditions, is malignant transformation. The major risk factors for development of GTD are maternal age older than 35 years and a history of GTD. Clinically, these patients often complain of vaginal bleeding and pelvic pain. On examination, they are often found to have an enlarged uterus and hyperemesis. Vaginal examination may show passage of hydrops vesicles.[34–38] Ultrasonography of a complete mole shows a central heterogeneous mass, with numerous discrete anechoic spaces. This finding corresponds to diffuse hydatidiform swelling of the hydropic chorionic villi. In years past, the term snowstorm was used to describe the appearance of molar pregnancies on ultrasonography. As technology has advanced, the description of a molar pregnancy on ultrasonography has changed. With the enhanced resolution that is achievable on newer ultrasound machines, molar pregnancies appear more like hypoechoic clusters of villi within the hyperechoic uterine tissue (**Fig. 14**).

Providers should be aware that the diagnosis of a partial mole is challenging with bedside ultrasonography. Partial moles show focal anechoic spaces within the placenta, often in the setting of a viable, but growth-restricted, fetus.[39] Immediate obstetric consultation is warranted if bedside ultrasonography detects any cystic mass or abnormal tissue in the uterus.

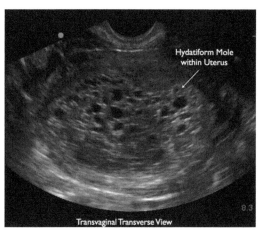

Fig. 14. Molar pregnancy.

EMERGENCY ULTRASONOGRAPHY IN THE GYNECOLOGIC PATIENT

A multitude of gynecologic diseases can be detected by bedside ultrasonography. For all of the following diseases, endocavitary ultrasonography is recommended, although, in each case, if the finding is large enough, it may be seen on transabdominal ultrasonography as well. The following section reviews ovarian disease followed by select uterine diseases.

OVARIAN CYSTS

Ovarian cysts can be simple (functional), complex, dermoid, or chocolate cysts (**Fig. 15**).

Simple cysts include follicular cysts, corpus luteum cysts, and theca lutein cysts. These cysts generally have thin walls, measure 3 to 8 cm in diameter, and are unilocular.[40] If a cyst larger than 3 cm is diagnosed on bedside ultrasonography, a 6-week follow-up scan should be obtained to ensure resolution.

Complex cysts are ones that show septations on ultrasonography, are irregular in terms of wall thickening (areas of the cyst wall are >2–3 mm), or have areas of shadowing echodensity.[40] These patients should be referred to gynecology urgently for workup of a possible malignancy, although during the reproductive years most of these masses are usually benign.

Dermoid cysts, also termed mature cystic teratomas, are the most common ovarian neoplasm and the most common benign germ cell tumor. These germ cell tumors consist of tissue derived from all 3 germ cell layers, and therefore often contain teeth, hair, and fat. On ultrasonography, they appear as a hyperechoic solid mass with fluid-fluid levels seen within the structure (**Fig. 16**).[7,40] Computed tomography or magnetic resonance imaging is often required for confirmation of this diagnosis. Again, urgent gynecology consultation is warranted.

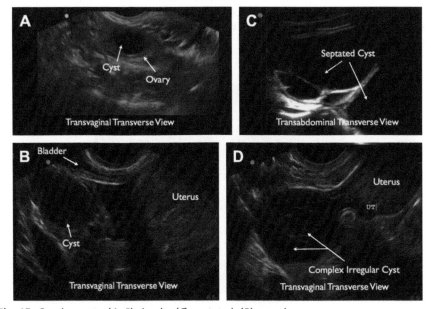

Fig. 15. Ovarian cysts: (*A, B*) simple; (*C*) septated; (*D*) complex.

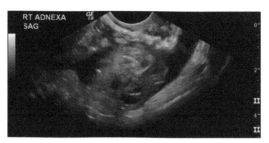

Fig. 16. Ultrasonography of a mature cystic teratoma. (*Courtesy of* Dr Teresa Wu, Maricopa Medical Center, University of Arizona, College of Medicine–Phoenix, AZ.)

Chocolate cysts are seen in patients with endometriosis. Endometrial tissue that has implanted on the ovary becomes covered with thick and fibrotic adhesions. This structure, when enlarged because of hormone-dependent changes, appears filled with homogenous hypoechoic low-level echoes.[40] Pathology specimens show chocolate-colored partially liquid material, which is why they are termed chocolate cysts.

OVARIAN TORSION

Ovarian torsion is a rare phenomenon, which is often difficult to diagnose based on symptoms and physical examination findings alone. Ovarian torsion accounts for only 3% of emergent gynecologic surgeries.[40] Primary ovarian torsion is seen more often in children, whereas in reproductive-aged women, torsion occurs because of the presence of an ovarian mass, such as a large functional cyst, complex cyst, polycystic ovarian syndrome, or ovarian hyperstimulation syndrome.[40] Torsion of the ovary results from the ovary twisting, either partially or completely, on its axis around the fallopian tube. Although ultrasonography is the recommended imaging modality, it is important to remember that ultrasonography is not 100% sensitive for this diagnosis.[40,41] This situation is because the arterial blood supply of the ovary comes from both the uterine and the ovarian arteries. Thus, the classic findings of ovarian enlargement caused by edema from the venous and lymphatic congestion produced by torsion may not be present if there is still some patent blood flow from another arterial source (**Fig. 17**).

Other findings suggestive of ovarian torsion include the presence of numerous enlarged follicles, formed by leaking of fluid into the follicles after edema has set in, and multiple engorged blood vessels in the periphery.[40] These findings are less common, and are challenging to discern as representative of torsion, because often women in whom torsion is being considered already have enlarged follicles or cysts in the ovary. For these reasons, experts recommend obtaining comprehensive ultrasonography via the radiology department to evaluate for the presence of ovarian torsion in high-risk scenarios. Experts also recommend obtaining a simultaneous obstetrics consultation if there is high clinical suspicion for ovarian torsion, even in the setting of negative ultrasonography. As mentioned earlier, ultrasonography is not 100% sensitive for ovarian torsion, and the findings of ovarian engorgement and complete absence of blood flow are late sonographic signs of an already ischemic ovary.

TOA, HYDROSALPINX, AND PYOSALPINX

Bedside ultrasonography is useful for the evaluation of ascending spread of infection in patients with cervicitis. As the infection ascends the genital tract, complications such as hydrosalpinx, pyosalpinx, or TOA can occur (**Fig. 18**).

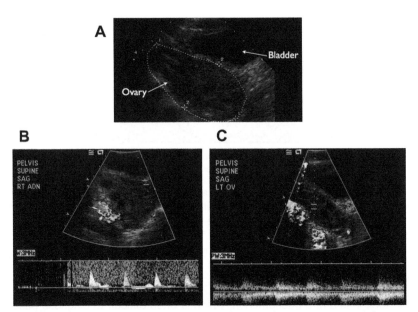

Fig. 17. Ovarian torsion: (A) enlarged ovary (8 × 4 cm); (B) abnormal arterial flow present only in periphery with decreased diastolic flow; (C) normal left ovary with normal systolic and diastolic flow. (*Courtesy of* Beverley Newman, MD and Bo Yoon Ha, MD, Stanford, CA.)

These findings are easily appreciated on endocavitary ultrasonography and may guide decisions for duration of antibiotic therapy, inpatient versus outpatient treatment, and prognosis. Hydrosalpinx is diagnosed when the fallopian tubes measure more than 5 mm in diameter and are filled with hypoechoic fluid.[40,42] In pyosalpinx, the fluid filling the fallopian tubes appears hyperechoic or echodense and heterogeneous, and the tube itself appears thicker in diameter than in hydrosalpinx.[40] An adnexal mass that is heterogeneous and tender suggests a TOA. Application of color Doppler over the TOA shows increased blood flow in the periphery, suggesting acute inflammation.

UTERINE LEIOMYOMAS

Leiomyomas, or fibroids, are commonly encountered smooth muscle tumors. It is estimated that approximately 25% of women older than 30 years have 1 fibroid.[40] The

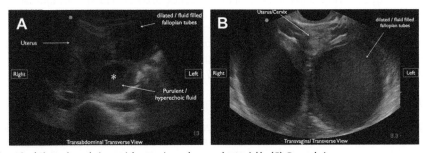

Fig. 18. (A) Hydrosalpinx with ovarian abscess (*asterisk*). (B) Pyosalpinx.

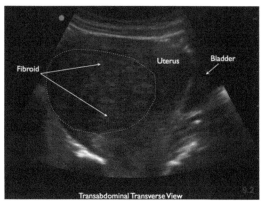

Fig. 19. Uterine fibroid.

location of these tumors can vary, from subserosal to submucosal to intramucosal. They may be found in the cervix or uterus, or attached to the uterus by a pedicle. Given their prevalence, it is helpful for providers to be familiar with their appearance (**Fig. 19**).

Fibroids can cause pelvic pressure and pain, as well as vaginal bleeding. On ultrasonography, central hypoechoic necrosis of the fibroid may be noted. Gynecology referral is warranted in cases of severe bleeding or pain.

IUD ASSESSMENT

An IUD is a metal T-shaped device inserted into the uterine fundus as a form of birth control. A string attached to the bottom of the device protrudes from the cervix, and usually enables the patient and provider to confirm the location of the IUD. However, migration of the IUD frequently occurs, and can result in complications ranging from uterine perforation to displacement into the endometrial canal to expulsion from the uterus.[13] Localization of the IUD on bedside ultrasonography is therefore an important and easily acquired skill. The metal structure of the IUD appears highly echogenic on ultrasonography and gives off reverberation, or ring-down, artifact (**Fig. 20**).

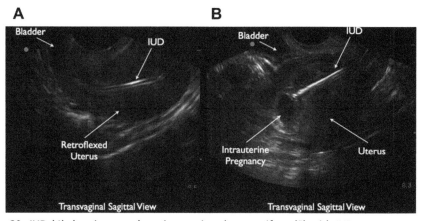

Fig. 20. IUD (A) showing reverberation or ring-down artifact; (B) with IUP.

Newer IUD models that are not made of metal can still be seen within the uterus. The nonmetallic IUDs appear as a hyperechoic structure with significant acoustic shadowing, but no ring-down artifact. Using the endocavitary probe, the surrounding uterine wall can be inspected, and the IUD placement can be determined.[43]

SUMMARY

Ultrasonography is the ideal diagnostic modality for evaluation of the female pelvis. In this article, the basic technique of performing transabdominal and transvaginal pelvic ultrasonography in the acute care setting is reviewed. After reading this article, providers should be comfortable assessing the uterus for a normal IUP, as well as recognizing various abnormalities, ranging from ectopic pregnancy to fetal bradycardia. Providers should also be comfortable evaluating the ovaries and fallopian tubes using bedside ultrasonography. Pelvic ultrasonography can be used at the bedside to accurately diagnose a range of common and uncommon condition, to expedite patient care, and to improve patient satisfaction.

REFERENCES

1. McRae A, Murray H, Edmonds M. Diagnostic accuracy and clinical usefulness of emergency department targeted ultrasonography in the evaluation of first-trimester pelvic pain and bleeding: a systematic review. CJEM 2009;11(4): 355–64.
2. Shalev E, Yarom I, Bustan M, et al. Transvaginal sonography as the ultimate diagnostic tool for the management of ectopic pregnancy: experience with 840 cases. Fertil Steril 1998;69(1):62–5.
3. Kirk E, Papageorghiou AT, Condous G, et al. The diagnostic effectiveness of an initial transvaginal scan in detecting ectopic pregnancy. Hum Reprod 2007; 22(11):2824–8. http://dx.doi.org/10.1093/humrep/dem283.
4. Mateer JR, Valley VT, Aiman EJ, et al. Outcome analysis of a protocol including bedside endovaginal sonography in patients at risk for ectopic pregnancy. Ann Emerg Med 1996;27(3):283–9.
5. Griffin Y, Sudigali V, Jacques A. Radiology of benign disorders of menstruation. Semin Ultrasound CT MR 2010;31(5):414–32. http://dx.doi.org/10.1053/j.sult. 2010.08.001.
6. Jang TB, Ruggeri W, Dyne P, et al. Learning curve of emergency physicians using emergency bedside sonography for symptomatic first-trimester pregnancy. J Ultrasound Med 2010;29(10):1423–8.
7. Brown DL, Dudiak KM, Laing FC. Adnexal masses: US characterization and reporting. Radiology 2010;254(2):342–54. http://dx.doi.org/10.1148/radiol. 09090552.
8. Dart RG. Role of pelvic ultrasonography in evaluation of symptomatic first-trimester pregnancy. Ann Emerg Med 1999;33(3):310–20.
9. Durham B, Lane B, Burbridge L, et al. Pelvic ultrasound performed by emergency physicians for the detection of ectopic pregnancy in complicated first-trimester pregnancies. Ann Emerg Med 1997;29(3):338–47.
10. Kirk E, Papageorghiou AT, Condous G, et al. The accuracy of first trimester ultrasound in the diagnosis of hydatidiform mole. Ultrasound Obstet Gynecol 2007; 29(1):70–5. http://dx.doi.org/10.1002/uog.3875.
11. Fowler DJ, Lindsay I, Seckl MJ, et al. Histomorphometric features of hydatidiform moles in early pregnancy: relationship to detectability by ultrasound examination.

Ultrasound Obstet Gynecol 2007;29(1):76–80. http://dx.doi.org/10.1002/uog. 3880.

12. Johns J, Greenwold N, Buckley S, et al. A prospective study of ultrasound screening for molar pregnancies in missed miscarriages. Ultrasound Obstet Gynecol 2005;25(5):493–7. http://dx.doi.org/10.1002/uog.1888.

13. Boortz HE, Margolis DJ, Ragavendra N, et al. Migration of intrauterine devices: radiologic findings and implications for patient care. Radiographics 2012;32(2): 335–52. http://dx.doi.org/10.1148/rg.322115068.

14. Cacciatore B, Tiitinen A, Stenman UH, et al. Normal early pregnancy: serum hCG levels and vaginal ultrasonography findings. Br J Obstet Gynaecol 1990;97(10): 899–903.

15. Bradley WG, Fiske CE, Filly RA. The double sac sign of early intrauterine pregnancy: use in exclusion of ectopic pregnancy. Radiology 1982;143(1): 223–6.

16. Yeh HC, Goodman JD, Carr L, et al. Intradecidual sign: a US criterion of early intrauterine pregnancy. Radiology 1986;161(2):463–7.

17. Nyberg DA, Laing FC, Filly RA, et al. Ultrasonographic differentiation of the gestational sac of early intrauterine pregnancy from the pseudogestational sac of ectopic pregnancy. Radiology 1983;146(3):755–9.

18. Nyberg DA, Filly RA, Filho DL, et al. Abnormal pregnancy: early diagnosis by US and serum chorionic gonadotropin levels. Radiology 1986;158(2):393–6.

19. Bailey C, Carnell J, Vahidnia F, et al. Accuracy of emergency physicians using ultrasound measurement of crown-rump length to estimate gestational age in pregnant women. Am J Emerg Med 2012;30(8):1627–9. http://dx.doi.org/10. 1016/j.ajem.2011.12.002.

20. Shah S, Teismann N, Zaia B, et al. Accuracy of emergency physicians using ultrasound to determine gestational age in pregnant women. Am J Emerg Med 2010;28(7):834–8. http://dx.doi.org/10.1016/j.ajem.2009.07.024.

21. Hadlock FP, Shah YP, Kanon DJ, et al. Fetal crown-rump length: reevaluation of relation to menstrual age (5–18 weeks) with high-resolution real-time US. Radiology 1992;182(2):501–5.

22. Hitty LS, Altman DG, Henderson A, et al. Charts of fetal size: 4. femur length. Br J Obstet Gynaecol 1994;101(2):132–5.

23. Farrant P, Meire HB. Ultrasound measurement of fetal limb lengths. Br J Radiol 1981;54(644):660–4.

24. Saraiya M, Berg CJ, Shulman H, et al. Estimates of the annual number of clinically recognized pregnancies in the United States, 1981–1991. Am J Epidemiol 1999; 149(11):1025–9.

25. Ectopic pregnancy mortality–Florida, 2009–2010. Available at: http://www.cdc. gov/mmwr/preview/mmwrhtml/mm6106a2.htm. Accessed January 23, 2013.

26. Braffman BH, Coleman BG, Ramchandani P, et al. Emergency department screening for ectopic pregnancy: a prospective US study. Radiology 1994; 190(3):797–802.

27. Barnhart KT. Clinical practice. Ectopic pregnancy. N Engl J Med 2009;361(4): 379–87. http://dx.doi.org/10.1056/NEJMcp0810384.

28. Frates MC, Laing FC. Sonographic evaluation of ectopic pregnancy: an update. AJR Am J Roentgenol 1995;165(2):251–9.

29. Moore C, Todd WM, O'Brien E, et al. Free fluid in Morison's pouch on bedside ultrasound predicts need for operative intervention in suspected ectopic pregnancy. Acad Emerg Med 2007;14(8):755–8. http://dx.doi.org/10.1197/j.aem. 2007.04.010.

30. Reece EA, Petrie RH, Sirmans MF, et al. Combined intrauterine and extrauterine gestations: a review. Am J Obstet Gynecol 1983;146(3):323–30.

31. Tal J, Haddad S, Gordon N, et al. Heterotopic pregnancy after ovulation induction and assisted reproductive technologies: a literature review from 1971 to 1993. Fertil Steril 1996;66(1):1–12.

32. Cheng PJ, Chueh HY, Qiu JT. Heterotopic pregnancy in a natural conception cycle presenting as hematometra. Obstet Gynecol 2004;104(5):1195–8. http://dx.doi.org/10.1097/01.AOG.0000142698.17433.cd.

33. Seeber BE, Barnhart KT. Suspected ectopic pregnancy. Obstet Gynecol 2006;107(2):399–413. http://dx.doi.org/10.1097/01.AOG.0000198632.15229.be.

34. Berkowitz RS, Tuncer ZS, Bernstein MR, et al. Management of gestational trophoblastic diseases: subsequent pregnancy experience. Semin Oncol 2000;27(6):678–85.

35. Lorigan PC, Sharma S, Bright N, et al. Characteristics of women with recurrent molar pregnancies. Gynecol Oncol 2000;78(3):288–92. http://dx.doi.org/10.1006/gyno.2000.5871.

36. Bagshawe KD, Dent J, Webb J. Hydatidiform mole in England and Wales 1973–83. Lancet 1986;2(8508):673–7.

37. Berkowitz RS, Im SS, Bernstein MR, et al. Gestational trophoblastic disease. subsequent pregnancy outcome, including repeat molar pregnancy. J Reprod Med 1998;43(1):81–6.

38. Sand PK, Lurain JR, Brewer JI. Repeat gestational trophoblastic disease. Obstet Gynecol 1984;63(2):140–4.

39. Fine C, Bundy AL, Berkowitz RS, et al. Sonographic diagnosis of partial hydatidiform mole. Obstet Gynecol 1989;73(3):414–8.

40. Cosby KS, Kendall JL. Practical guide to emergency ultrasound. Philadelphia: Lippincott Williams & Wilkins; 2006. p. 161–83.

41. Mashiach R, Melamed N, Gilad N, et al. Sonographic diagnosis of ovarian torsion: accuracy and predictive factors. J Ultrasound Med 2011;30(9):1205–10.

42. Guerriero S, Ajossa S, Lai MP, et al. Transvaginal ultrasonography associated with colour Doppler energy in the diagnosis of hydrosalpinx. Hum Reprod 2000;15(7):1568–72.

43. Palo P. Transabdominal and transvaginal ultrasound detection of levonorgestrel IUD in the uterus. Acta Obstet Gynecol Scand 1997;76(3):244–7.

Bedside Ocular Ultrasound

Pedro J. Roque, MD[a],*, Nicholas Hatch, MD[a], Laurel Barr, MD[a],
Teresa S. Wu, MD[b]

KEYWORDS

- Ocular ultrasound • Eye ultrasound • Bedside eye ultrasound
- Bedside ocular ultrasound • Retinal detachment • Globe rupture • Lens dislocation
- Vitreous hemorrhage

KEY POINTS

- Perform an ocular ultrasound on any patient suspected of having ocular trauma, visual changes, eye pain, or a suspected foreign body.
- Use the examination function for nerve, small parts, or ocular settings and increase the gain to evaluate for subtle posterior chamber findings.
- Dynamic extraocular movements during the ocular ultrasound may help unveil subtle pathology, such as a small retinal tear or vitreous hemorrhage, and should be included in the ultrasound examination if possible.

INTRODUCTION

The eye is a fluid-filled structure that lies superficially within the orbit, making it one of the easiest objects to visualize with ultrasound examination. Although CT and MRI are invaluable to the diagnosis of many orbital pathologies, they lack the immediacy and the simplicity of ultrasound and cannot provide real-time images. Ultrasound is, therefore, more effective at the diagnosis of various tissue diagnoses, such as retinal detachment and vitreous hemorrhage, both of which are difficult to visualize with conventional static images of CT or MRI.[1] Furthermore, ultrasound allows practitioners to evaluate the structures of the globe in a dynamic fashion at the bedside, even in situations where orbital swelling, trauma, and patient cooperation inhibit direct visualization of the eye for a traditional ocular examination.

EYE AND ORBIT ANATOMY

In order to interpret the images of a pathologic eye, it is vital to understand the anatomy and the points of firm attachment of the vitreous, retina, and choroid in a normal

---

[a] Department of Emergency Medicine, Maricopa Medical Center, 2601 East Roosevelt Street, Phoenix, AZ 85008, USA; [b] Department of Emergency Medicine, Maricopa Medical Center, University of Arizona, School of Medicine-Phoenix, 2601 East Roosevelt Street, Phoenix, AZ 85008, USA
* Corresponding author.
E-mail address: pjroquemd@gmail.com

Crit Care Clin 30 (2014) 227–241
http://dx.doi.org/10.1016/j.ccc.2013.10.007   criticalcare.theclinics.com

eye (**Box 1**, **Fig. 1**). The eyeball lies surrounded by fat but separated from it by a membranous sac, termed Tenon capsule. Its attachments include the corneoscleral junction and the optic nerve. This sac is in turn pierced by the extraocular muscle tendons. On ultrasound evaluation, the surrounding facial bones appear as bright reflectors with deep posterior shadowing.[2,3] The eyeball contains 2 major fluid-filled compartments called the anterior chamber and the posterior chamber (see **Fig. 1**).[1] Echolucent aqueous humor fills the anterior chamber, and vitreous humor fills the posterior chamber. The normal anterior and posterior chambers of the eye should be completely anechoic (see **Fig. 1**).[1]

Sclera and Cornea

The outer wall of the eyeball consists of 3 layers. The outermost layer is tough and fibrous and contains the sclera and the cornea, both of which are mostly avascular. **Fig. 1** illustrates the cuplike extension of the sclera as it extends from the dural sheath of the optic nerve. The sclera bulges forward anteriorly, thereby forming the cornea, which overlies the entire anterior chamber (see **Fig. 1**). The cornea appears as a thin hyperechoic structure attached to the sclera at the periphery.[1] The corneoscleral junction contains 2 sinuses called the canal of Schlemm at the periphery of the anterior chamber. This canal is responsible for the drainage of aqueous humor, which then communicates with the anterior scleral veins.

Choroid, Ciliary Body, and Iris

The choroid, ciliary body, and iris (like the sclera) are cuplike extensions of the arachnoid and pia mater layers of the optic nerve posteriorly (see **Fig. 1**). The choroid layer begins as the optic nerve meets the posterior chamber and travels anteriorly toward the anterior chamber. It turns into the ciliary bodies bilaterally at the junction of the anterior/posterior chambers and the vitreous, which are responsible for pupil dilation and constriction. The choroid is firmly attached to the sclera throughout, with the firmest points of attachment the scleral spur and the exit foramina of the vortex veins (see **Fig. 1**).[1] The choroid is an avascular layer that is of lower reflectivity than the retina or the sclera on ultrasound. The iris is the last segment of the choroid anteriorly acting as a contractile diaphragm situated directly anterior to the lens. It is

---

Box 1
Review of the important anatomic considerations, including the key firm attachment points of the eye critical to understanding ocular pathology

The inner wall of the orbit consists of the retina, choroid, and the sclera (anteriorly to posteriorly).

The firm attachment points of the various layers of the inner orbit are critical to the understanding of ocular detachments.

The posterior layers of the eye consist of the retina and the choroid, bound by the sclera.

The 2 most important attachments of the choroid are the scleral spur and the exit foramina of the vortex veins.

The 2 most important attachments of the retina are the optic nerve head and the ora serrata.

The 2 most important attachments of the vitreous are the pars plana and optic disc.

Elevated optic nerve sheath diameter is associated with an elevation of intracranial pressure. A normal optic nerve sheath diameter is <5 mm (adults), <4.5 mm (children 1–15 years old), and <4.0 mm (infants <1 years old).

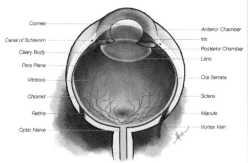
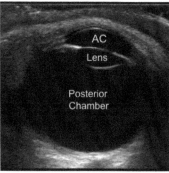

Fig. 1. (*Left*) Image medical illustration of normal eye anatomy. (*Right*) Image of an ocular ultrasound illustrating the normal anterior and posterior chambers of the eye. AC, anterior chamber. (*Courtesy of* [*left*] Nicholas Hatch, MD, Phoenix, AZ; and [*right*] T. Wu, MD, Phoenix, AZ.)

approximately 1 mm in thickness and obscures the anterior lens surface on ultrasound scans.[1] The iris also partially separates the anterior chamber from the posterior chamber of the eye.

Retina

The retina is the innermost membrane of the eyeball, composed entirely of nervous membrane tissue. It is the neural sensory stratum of the globe. Its anterior surface is in direct contact with the vitreous body and its posterior surface is strongly adhered to the choroid with 2 important firm attachment points: the optic nerve head and the ora serrata.[1] These are the 2 firmest points of attachment of the choroid to the retina (see **Fig. 1**). The ora serrata represents the junction of the end of the retina and the pars plana, as illustrated in **Fig. 2**. The optic disc has a diameter of approximately 1.5 mm and is situated slightly above the level of the posterior pole. It is the important site of entry for the retinal arteries and the exit point for the retinal nerves and veins.[1] On B-mode ultrasound, the retina should be completely adherent to the posterior globe and there should be no separation visualized during the scan (see **Fig. 2**).[1]

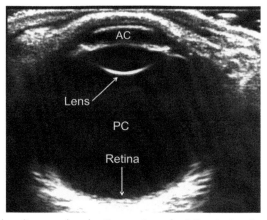

Fig. 2. Normal ocular ultrasound and retina on B-mode. AC, anterior chamber; PC, posterior chamber. (*Courtesy of* T. Wu, MD, Phoenix, AZ.)

Refractory Media

The refractory media of the eyeball include the cornea, aqueous humor, lens, and vitreous body. The aqueous humor consists of a saline solution that is secreted into the posterior chamber from the iris and ciliary bodies and travels into the anterior chamber through the pupil.[1] The lens appears as a hyperechoic reflector, which is biconcave and enclosed in a transparent elastic capsule. The central posterior layer of the lens gives off a faint echo, giving rise to a fine curved line on ultrasound images (see **Fig. 2**).[2] The largest fluid-filled cavity in the eyeball is the vitreous body comprising approximately 80% of the total globe volume.[2] It lies behind the posterior chamber and is composed of a gel-like substance containing mucopolysaccharides and water. It is attached firmly at the optic disc and the pars plana.[2] It otherwise lies in free contact with the retina. Normal vitreous gel is anechoic (black on ultrasound); however, it is sometimes seen undulating off the retina posteriorly when scanning during dynamic extraocular movements (see **Fig. 2**).[2]

Optic Nerve and Ophthalmic Vessels

The optic nerve, sheath, and vessels may be seen posteriorly on ultrasound examination traveling toward the optic chiasm. On ultrasound examination, the nerve appears mostly hypoechoic with low internal reflectivity, flanked by a more echogenic nerve sheath at the periphery (**Fig. 3**).[4]

By convention, measurements of the optic nerve sheath diameter are made 3-mm posterior to the globe (see **Fig. 3**). A normal optic nerve sheath diameter in adults is defined as less than 5 mm. In children between 1 and 15 years of age, a normal optic nerve sheath diameter should be less than 4.5 mm, and in infants under 1 year of age, it should be less then 4 mm.[4–6] Measurement by ultrasound of the optic nerve sheath

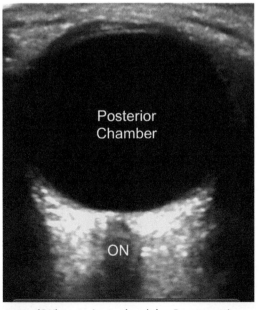

Fig. 3. Normal optic nerve (ON) posterior to the globe. By convention, measurements of the optic nerve sheath diameter are made 3 mm posterior to the globe. (*Courtesy of* T. Wu, MD, Phoenix, AZ.)

diameter is clinically important because the inner layer of the optic nerve sheath is an extension of the subarachnoid space stemming from the central nervous system. It distends in response to elevations in intracranial pressure from trauma, mass effect, or even malignant hypertension.[4–7]

Color Doppler ultrasound can also be used to identify the arterial and venous structures within the eye. The largest vascular structure in the eye is the ophthalmic artery, which runs parallel to the optic nerve.[2] The central retinal arteries and veins can be detected using bedside ocular ultrasound. They both run together in the anterior portion of the optic nerve shadow. They are easily distinguished using pulse wave Doppler and color Doppler examination of the posterior orbit.[8]

OCULAR ULTRASOUND EXAMINATION TECHNIQUE
Patient Positioning

As with most ultrasound examinations, the ultrasound machine is placed on the patient's right so that the practitioner can scan with the right hand. Patient positioning varies depending on a patient's clinical history. Trauma patients with potential spine injuries may have to remain lying supine, whereas others may be able to sit partially or completely upright for the examination. A high-frequency linear array transducer in the 7.5-MHz to 15-MHz frequency range is preferred for this examination because superficial structures are best visualized with higher-frequency probes. The higher-frequency transducer allows for a sharper image; however, its limited penetration can reduce visualization of retro-orbital structures. Some ultrasound machines are also equipped with color or spectral Doppler technology, allowing for the visualization of orbital vasculature during the scan.

Technique

Depending on the ultrasound machine used, either the small parts, nerve, or ocular/ophthalmic settings can be used. The gel used for an ocular ultrasound examination does not need to be sterile. In most situations, it is recommended that individualized gel packets (eg, Surgilube) be used for the ocular ultrasound because the gel is water based and bacteriostatic. To begin the scan, place a large amount of gel over the patient's closed eyelid and fill the entire preorbital space. The goal is to apply enough gel so that the transducer can float over the layer of gel and never come in direct contact with the patient's eyelid (**Fig. 4**). This is critical in the event of a possible ruptured

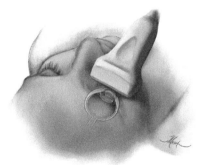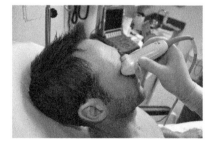

Fig. 4. (*Left*) An artistic representation of an eye ultrasound performed in the transverse plane along with the relevant eye anatomy deep to the probe. (*Right*) Image showing a sonographer performing an ocular ultrasound in the transverse plane. (*Courtesy of* [*left*] N. Hatch, MD, Phoenix, AZ; and [*right*] T. Cook, MD, Columbia, SC.)

globe, where any pressure transferred to the globe could potentially cause vitreous extrusion.

Alternatively, prior to beginning the scan, a thin piece of Tegaderm can be applied to the closed eyelid before gel is applied. The thin Tegaderm serves to shield the patient's eye from any exposure to the gel being applied. Ensure that the Tegaderm is pressed securely to the closed eyelid and that all air bubbles are eliminated before applying gel over the Tegaderm barrier. Air pockets can produce artifacts that may interfere with interpretation of the scan.

During the ocular scan, the transducer should be oriented with the indicator pointing toward the top of the patient's head for longitudinal views and toward the patient's right for transverse views. This allows for proper identification of the nasal and temporal portions of the eye during image review (**Fig. 5**).

The sonographer must take care to maintain a separation between the probe and the eyelid to avoid placing any direct pressure onto the orbit. Simply suspending the transducer over a patient's eye produces lower-quality images and eventually leads to increased pressure over the eyeball as the practitioner's arm fatigues. By stabilizing the hypothenar eminence and small finger over the subject's nose or midface, the practitioner can avoid arm fatigue and obtain higher-quality images.[2]

Once the probe is positioned appropriately, the next step is to adjust the gain on the ultrasound machine. A normal gain should be used for the initial evaluation. The gain can later be increased to look for more subtle pathology, such as retinal detachment or vitreous hemorrhage. Ultrasound imaging almost always occurs in 2 planes, allowing reconstructing a 3-D mental image of the target structure being scanned. It is important to sweep the transducer from side to side in both planes in order to obtain the greatest amount of information. A cooperative patient can also aid in the ultrasound examination by moving his eyes up and down and then side to side, while maintaining a closed eyelid. This eye movement may unmask subtle pathology, such as small retinal tears or subtle vitreous hemorrhage.

The posterior orbital structures can also be easily visualized by using bedside ocular ultrasound. Pathology, such as retrobulbar hematoma, elevated optic nerve sheath diameters, ocular abscesses, central retinal artery occlusion, and central retinal vein occlusion, can be identified if the space behind the globe is fully evaluated (**Box 2**).

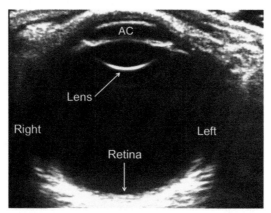

Fig. 5. Ocular ultrasound orientation. Note that the probe is positioned in a transverse fashion with the indicator pointing toward the patient's right. AC, anterior chamber. (*Courtesy of* T. Wu, MD, Phoenix, AZ)

> **Box 2**
> **Review of patient positioning and ocular ultrasound techniques**
>
> Always place the ultrasound on the right side of the patient and orient the probe so that the indicator is pointing either toward the patient's head or toward the right side.
>
> Minimize the amount of pressure placed on the eyelid and globe during the scan.
>
> Set the examination mode to nerve, small parts, or an ocular setting.
>
> Start with a medium amount of gain and then increase the gain to evaluate for subtle findings.
>
> Fan through all transverse and longitudinal planes in order to get a good 3-D mental image of the orbit.

EMERGENT OCULAR ABNORMALITIES
Retinal Detachment

Bedside ultrasound allows for quick and accurate diagnosis of retinal detachment so that treatment may be instituted as rapidly as possible. Recently, Blaivas and colleagues[9] published a study assessing the accuracy of ocular ultrasonography in the emergency department.[10] This study showed that 60 of 61 intraocular diseases, including 9 retinal detachments, were accurately diagnosed by emergency practitioners trained in ocular ultrasound.[9] Shinar and colleagues[10] conducted a prospective observational study where emergency physicians, after a 30-minute training session, attempted to detect retinal detachment using ocular ultrasound. Emergency physicians achieved 97% sensitivity and 92% specificity on 92 examinations (29 retinal detachments).

Retinal detachment occurs on a continuum from small retinal tears to complete retinal detachments. Retinal detachments appear on ultrasound as highly reflective membranes floating in the substance of the vitreous body. During the ocular ultrasound, if a patient moves the eye, the detached retina can be seen floating and moving within the vitreous body. The firm anatomic attachments of the retina, at the ora serrata and the optic nerve head, ensure that the detachment does not extend past these sites (**Fig. 6**). A completely detached retina is still attached to the optic nerve head posteriorly and the ora serrata anteriorly, producing a classic V shape on ultrasound (see **Fig. 6**). Smaller retinal detachments may be seen as a linear hyperechoic structure floating off the posterior globe on bedside ultrasound (**Fig. 7**).

Retinal detachments must be differentiated from choroid detachments and vitreous detachments. The choroid layer lies one layer deep to the retina (see **Fig. 2**) and is, therefore, not in direct contact with the vitreous body. For this reason, choroidal detachments are usually thicker and remain fixed with eye movements during the ultrasound examination (**Fig. 8**). A vitreous detachment generally has a V-shaped appearance and appears within the vitreous body. Similar to choroid detachment, it does not change or undulate with eye movements.

Vitreous Hemorrhage

Vitreous hemorrhage frequently accompanies trauma; however, it can occur spontaneously. The presence of blood has a destructive effect on the vitreous gel structure leading to formations of echogenic opacities of varying sizes throughout the vitreous (**Fig. 9**).[1] The ultrasound images of vitreous hemorrhage ultimately depend on both the age and severity of the hemorrhage. Small vitreous hemorrhages may not be detected using the normal gain setting. They can sometimes be detected by increasing the gain of the ultrasound machine while having the patient perform eye movements to all

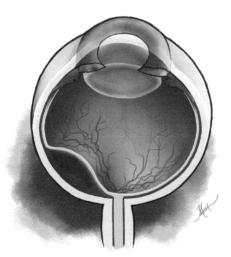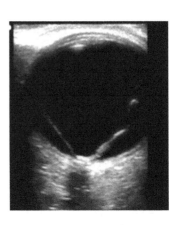

Fig. 6. (*Left*) Image of an illustration of a retinal detachment. (*Right*) Image of an ultrasound image of a complete retinal detachment. Note that the retina remains attached to its firm attachment points at the ora serrata bilaterally and the optic nerve head posteriorly producing the classic V shape on ultrasound. (*Courtesy of* [*left*] N. Hatch, MD, Phoenix, AZ; and [*right*] T. Cook, MD, Columbia, SC.)

4 quadrants. This eye movement enhances visualization of the hemorrhage as the hyperechoic particles of blood are seen swirling around in the vitreous (see **Fig. 9**). These opacities may also layer because gravity and gentle eye movements can bring them anteriorly for better visualization.

Lens Dislocation

Ectopia lentis, otherwise known as dislocation or malposition of the eye lens, can also be detected on bedside ultrasound. The most common cause of a lens dislocation is

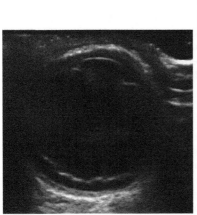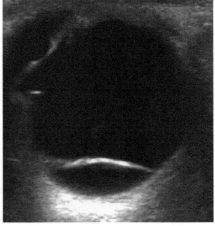

Fig. 7. Transverse ocular ultrasound images of retinal detachment. (*Courtesy of* T. Wu, MD, Phoenix, AZ.)

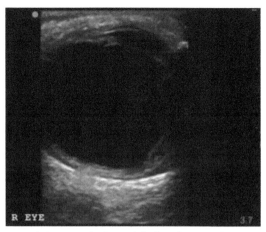

Fig. 8. Ocular ultrasound image of choroidal detachment. (*Courtesy of* T. Cook, MD, Columbia, SC.)

trauma.[11] Lens dislocation is easily visualized with ocular ultrasound when clinically significant (**Fig. 10**). There are 2 major types of lens dislocations: partial (subluxation) or complete. The key to the diagnosis lies with dynamic scanning. In a partial lens dislocation (subluxation), the lens moves independently of the intended extraocular movement. A complete lens dislocation shows the lens out of the lens patellar fossa and floating in the anterior chamber, in the vitreous humor, or over the retina (see **Fig. 10**).[11]

Globe Rupture

Globe perforation is typically secondary to traumatic injury. Sonographically, a ruptured globe shows an overall loss of ocular volume indicating the loss of intraocular pressure and vitreous humor, distorted size and shape of the vitreous chamber, and

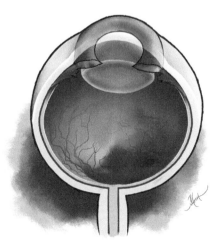
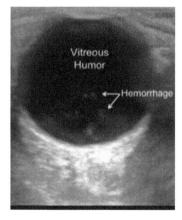

Fig. 9. (*Left*) Image showing a medical illustration of vitreous hemorrhage. (*Right*) Image showing the ultrasonographic appearance of vitreous hemorrhage. (*Courtesy of* [*left*] N. Hatch, MD, Phoenix, AZ; and [*right*] T. Wu, MD, Phoenix, AZ.)

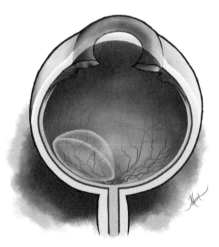

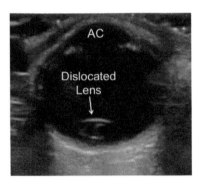

Fig. 10. (*Left*) Image of a medical illustration of lens dislocation. (*Right*) Image showing the ultrasonographic appearance of lens dislocation. AC, anterior chamber. (*Courtesy of* [*left*] N. Hatch, MD, Phoenix, AZ; and [*right*] T. Wu, MD, Phoenix, AZ.)

possibly intraocular air if there is communication with the ethmoid sinus (**Fig. 11**).[1] If there is significant intraorbital bleeding with the globe rupture, a hyperechoic and clotted vitreous chamber may be seen on bedside ultrasound (see **Fig. 11**).[1]

Small perforations of the globe may be missed if little vitreous is lost. For this reason, a thorough slit-lamp examination with fluorescein should also be completed if a globe rupture is suspected. A positive Seidel test is when the fluorescein strip turns pale on application to the corneal surface. This change in the color of the fluorescein strip is due to dilution of fluorescein caused by the aqueous leakage from the anterior chamber of the eye. A waterfall of fluorescein streaming down the cornea can also be seen

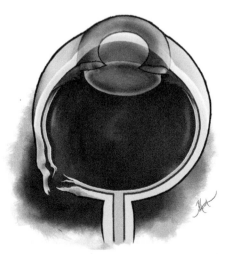

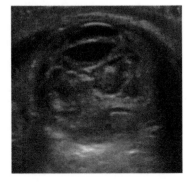

Fig. 11. (*Left*) Image is a medical illustration of globe rupture. (*Right*) Image showing the ultrasonographic appearance of globe rupture. (*Courtesy of* [*left*] N. Hatch, MD, Phoenix, AZ; and [*right*] T. Wu, MD, Phoenix, AZ.)

with perforation and aqueous humor leakage. In situations where a small globe rupture has sealed itself off, bedside ultrasound may be more sensitive for detecting globe injury than the Seidel test.

Optic Nerve Evaluation

Currently, the 3 methods of detecting increased intracranial pressure include a fundoscopic examination looking for papilledema; advanced imaging, such as a head CT or MRI; and direct intrathecal intracranial pressure monitoring. Patients with altered level of consciousness suffering from elevated intracranial pressure benefit from a rapid, effective, noninvasive, and portable evaluation for the detection of increased intracranial pressure. The correlation between optic nerve sheath diameter and elevated intracranial pressure has been well established.[4–6] A normal optic nerve sheath diameter in adults is defined as less than 5 mm. In children between 1 and 15 years of age, a normal optic nerve sheath diameter should be less than 4.5 mm, and in infants under 1 year of age, it should be less then 4 mm.[4–6]

Because the optic nerve sheath is a direct extension of the subarachnoid space of the central nervous system, its diameter correlates directly with increased intracranial pressures. There has been recent interest in evaluating the optic nerve sheath diameter in hypertensive patients to determine if there are signs of increased intracranial pressure during suspected hypertensive urgencies or emergencies. Early diagnosis of acute intracranial hypertension in the hypertensive population would be extremely useful to the treating physicians because it would lead to earlier blood pressure treatment and improved outcomes. Recently, Roque and colleagues[7] conducted a prospective, observational study of patients to evaluate the association between optic nerve sheath diameter and blood pressure readings. Their study demonstrated that optic nerve sheath diameters are increased in symptomatic patients with a blood pressure greater than 166/82 mm Hg. Optic nerve ultrasounds can be used to assess for elevated intracranial pressure at the bedside in patients with hypertension, trauma, cerebral infection, edema, or intracranial hemorrhage (**Fig. 12**). Findings can be used to prompt early intervention and help guide treatment options.

Retrobulbar Hematoma

On bedside ultrasound, a retrobulbar hematoma is seen as a hypoechoic collection of fluid just posterior to the globe (**Fig. 13**). Bleeding and edema behind the orbit can result in a quick elevation of retro-orbital pressure and consequently diminished circulation, ischemia, and later necrosis of the optic nerve (orbital compartment syndrome) with irreversible blindness.[12,13] Without prompt intervention, permanent reduction in visual acuity can develop in as little time as 90 minutes.[12,13] In trauma patients, identifying retrobulbar hemorrhage can be challenging, especially in the context of extensive facial trauma and periorbital edema. Performing a quick bedside ultrasound evaluation of the retro-orbital space can lead to early diagnosis of a retrobulbar hematoma and prompt emergent treatment with a lateral canthotomy.

Intraocular Foreign Bodies

It is typically easy to identify the presence of an ocular foreign body, as long as it is not embedded in the posterior orbital fat. Although in some cases, an intraocular foreign body may be observed and monitored clinically, in most cases (>90%) the foreign body must be removed surgically.[14,15] Expeditious and accurate identification of intraocular foreign bodies can lead to early intervention and better outcomes for the patient. Traditionally, orbital CT without contrast has been used to evaluate patients

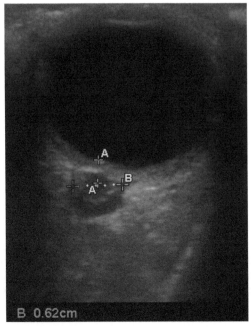

Fig. 12. Increased optic nerve sheath diameter in a patient with an intracranial hemorrhage. (*Courtesy of* T. Wu, MD, Phoenix, AZ.)

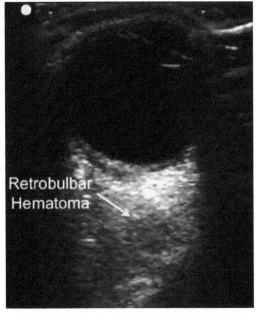

Fig. 13. Ocular ultrasound showing a retrobulbar hematoma. (*Courtesy of* T. Wu, MD, Phoenix, AZ.)

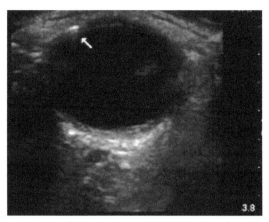

Fig. 14. *Arrow* pointing to metallic foreign body embedded in the eye. (*Courtesy of* T. Wu, MD, Phoenix, AZ.)

suspected of having an intraocular foreign body. Orbital CT may not be available in all instances, however, and it exposes patients to additional radiation risks.

Bedside ultrasound can be used to evaluate for the presence of intraocular foreign bodies. Metallic foreign bodies are the easiest to identify and appear as a bright, white, hyperechoic objects on ultrasound (**Fig. 14**). Larger metal objects may produce a ring down artifact farfield to the foreign body.

Color Doppler can also be used to help identify the presence of a foreign body. When color Doppler is applied over an echogenic foreign body, it produces a twinkling artifact. With color Doppler, this twinkling artifact appears as rapidly changing flashes of red and blue under the Doppler box.[16]

Periorbital Abscess

Bedside ocular ultrasound can also be used to evaluate for the presence of a periorbital abscess. A periorbital abscess appears as a distinct hypoechoic or heterogeneous collection of fluid lying just outside of the globe (**Fig. 15**). Application of color

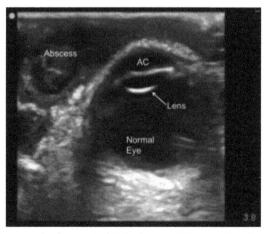

Fig. 15. Ocular ultrasound of a periorbital abscess. AC, anterior chamber. (*Courtesy of* T. Wu, MD, Phoenix, AZ.)

Doppler over the fluid collection shows enhanced color flow secondary to the inflamed tissue surrounding the abscess pocket. Ultrasound can be used to evaluate the size and depth of the abscess and to monitor for regression versus reaccumulation after treatment of the abscess.

SUMMARY

Bedside ocular ultrasound allows for the rapid, noninvasive, and dynamic examination of the eye and surrounding structures. Important data can be obtained in a matter of minutes without having to transfer or reposition patients. Pathologic findings can be detected without relying on patient cooperation or the ability to directly visualize the eye and posterior orbit. Practitioners performing ocular ultrasound examinations at the bedside can accurately detect a range of important eye disorders and rule out emergent conditions.

REFERENCES

1. Allan PL, Baxter GM, Weston MJ. Clinical ultrasound. 3rd edition. United Kingdom: Churchill Livingstone; 2011. p. 3–50, 938–64.
2. Ma OJ, Mateer JR, Blaivas M. Emergency ultrasound. 2nd edition. New York: McGraw Hill; 2008. p. 15–63.
3. Fielding JA. The assessment of ocular injury by ultrasound. Clin Radiol 2004;59: 301–12.
4. Newman W, Holliman A, Dutton G, et al. Measurement of optic nerve sheath diameter by ultrasound: a means of detecting acute raised intracranial pressure in hydrocephalus. Br J Ophthalmol 2002;86:1009–113.
5. Blaivas M, Theodoro D, Sierzenski P. Elevated intracranial pressure detected by bedside emergency ultrasonography of the optic nerve sheath. Acad Emerg Med 2003;10:376–81.
6. Tsung J, Blaivas M, Cooper A, et al. Rapid non-invasivemethod of detecting elevated intracranial pressure using ocular ultrasound: application to 3 cases of head trauma in the pediatric emergency department. Pediatr Emerg Care 2005;21:94–9.
7. Roque PJ, Wu TS, Barth L, et al. Optic nerve ultrasound for the detection of elevated intracranial pressure in the hypertensive patient. Am J Emerg Med 2012;30(8):1357–63.
8. Martini E, Guiducci M, Campi L, et al. Ocular blood flow evaluation in injured and heaalthy fellow eyes. Eur J Ophthalmol 2005;15:48–55.
9. Blaivas M, Theodoro D, Sierzenski P. A study of bedside ocular ultrasonography in the emergency department. Acad Emerg Med 2002;9:791–9.
10. Shinar Z, Chan L, Orlinsky M. Use of ocular ultrasound for the evaluation of retinal detachment. J Emerg Med 2011;40(1):53–7.
11. Jarrett WH. Dislocation of the lens. A study of 166 hospitalized cases. Arch Ophthalmol 1967;78:289–96.
12. Hislop WS, Dutton GN, Douglas PS. Treatment of retrobulbar haemorrhage in accident and emergency departments. Br J Oral Maxillofac Surg 1996;34:289–92.
13. Klenk G. Blindness caused by retrobulbar hemorrhage (orbital compartment syndrome). Orv Hetil 2010;151(38):1537–44.
14. Greven CM, Engelbrecht NE, Slusher MM, et al. Intraocular foreign bodies: management, prognostic factors, and visual outcomes. Ophthalmology 2000;107: 608–12.

15. Shiver SA, Lyon M, Blaivas M. Detection of metallic ocular foreign bodies with handheld sonography in a porcine model. J Ultrasound Med 2005;24(10): 1341–6.

16. Ustymowicz A, Krejza J, Mariak Z. Twinkling artifact in color Doppler imaging of the orbit. J Ultrasound Med 2002;21(5):559–63.

Bedside Musculoskeletal Ultrasonography

Mary J. Connell, MD[a,b,c,*], Teresa S. Wu, MD[c,d,e,f]

KEYWORDS

- Soft tissue ultrasound • Tendons • Muscles • Bones • Lipomas • Pilonidal cysts
- Cellulitis • Abscess

KEY POINTS

- Musculoskeletal sonography has been useful in point-of-care patient management for many years. Recent technologic advances have brought these applications into mainstream patient care for providers in many fields.
- The superficial location of many musculoskeletal structures lends itself to detailed and accurate depiction of anatomic and pathologic conditions affecting the musculoskeletal system.
- Structures easily portrayed on musculoskeletal ultrasound (US) images include subcutaneous fat, muscle, tendons, ligaments, and joints.
- The image resolution and diagnostic power of US exceeds that of CT and MRI of the musculoskeletal system for many conditions.
- Musculoskeletal US is indispensible in guiding many bedside procedures, including abscess diagnosis and drainage, vascular access, superficial biopsies, tendon and joint injections, and aspirations.

INTRODUCTION

The value of US in evaluating the musculoskeletal system has been recognized for more than 50 years.[1] Recent advances in technology have made this tool indispensable for evaluating patients with soft tissue and extremity complaints. There are many

Funding Sources: Nothing to disclose.
Conflict of Interest: Nothing to disclose.
[a] Maricopa Integrated Health Care System, 2601 East Roosevelt, Phoenix, AZ 85008, USA; [b] Diagnostic Radiology Residency, Maricopa Medical Center, 2601 East Roosevelt, Phoenix, AZ 85016, USA; [c] University of Arizona College of Medicine-Phoenix, 550 E. Van Buren, Phoenix, AZ 85004, USA; [d] Emergency Medicine Ultrasound Program & Fellowship, Maricopa Integrated Health Care System, 2601 East Roosevelt, Phoenix, AZ 85008, USA; [e] Simulation Based Training Program & Fellowship, Maricopa Integrated Health Care System, 2601 East Roosevelt, Phoenix, AZ 85008, USA; [f] Emergency Medicine Residency Program, Maricopa Medical Center, 2601 East Roosevelt, Phoenix, AZ 85016, USA
* Corresponding author. Department of Radiology, Maricopa Medical Center, 2601 East Roosevelt, Phoenix, AZ 85016.
E-mail address: mary_connell@dmgaz.org

benefits to adding US to the physical evaluation.[2,3] Portable, compact units allow physicians to scan patients at the bedside, and enable physicians to use US as an extension of the physical examination.

Using point-of-care US can expedite patient evaluation and treatment.[2,4,5] When a musculoskeletal issue is addressed, CT or MRI is commonly included in the evaluation. Bedside US allows physicians to diagnose common causes of musculoskeletal ailments in a matter of minutes and can be performed easily in patients who cannot be transported for CT or MRI. Furthermore, bedside US examinations can be repeated to monitor progression or resolution of the disease process without exposing patients to additional radiation.[4,5]

The natural resolution provided by US of the musculoskeletal system frequently often makes contrast-enhanced CT unnecessary. Although CT delivers exquisite detail of musculoskeletal pathology, a careful US of the region can deliver the same information in a faster and more cost-effective manner (**Fig. 1**).[2] Obtaining a contrast-enhanced musculoskeletal CT not only exposes patients to the risks of radiation but also requires intravenous insertion and laboratory analysis of renal function

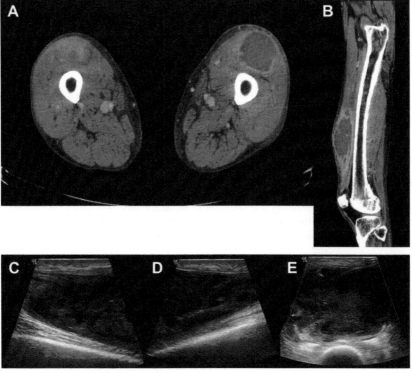

Fig. 1. Axial (*A*) and sagittal (*B*) contrast-enhanced CT images of an intramuscular abscess in the distal right quadriceps. C and D represent superior (*C*) and inferior (*D*) portions of the same area on a split screen gray scale ultrasound image, again demonstrating an intramuscular complex fluid collection anterior to the distal right femur. Note the muscle fibers separated by the fluid collection. (*E*) Short-axis US image of the same fluid collection, with color flow imaging, demonstrating mild peripheral hyperemia. This correlates with the CT finding of rim enhancement. Although the CT provides exquisite detail of the pathology, the same information is identified with US.

and puts patients at risk for contrast-induced reactions and side effects. MRIs are time and labor intensive and require hemodynamically stable and cooperative patients. Bedside US does not require any adjuncts and can provide adequate information to provide an accurate diagnosis.

US is well tolerated by most patients and can be tailored to a patient's complaint, physical examination findings, and tolerance of the examination. Awake and oriented patients are usually interested in their bedside US and can actively participate in the examination. Adding dynamic information, which may include gentle ballottement or having a patient move the extremity during the scan, adds important data typically not available by any other radiographic imaging modality.[5,6]

PROBE SELECTION

The key to obtaining useful information about most musculoskeletal pathology is using the highest frequency linear array transducer available. For most musculoskeletal imaging, an 8- to 14-MHz transducer should be used (**Fig. 2**).[3]

High-frequency transducers come in various shapes and footprints. Specialized transducers, such as the hockey stick footprint, can be useful during evaluation of smaller areas (**Fig. 3**).

Color flow or power Doppler imaging can be used to identify hyperemia or neovascularity within inflamed areas. In patients undergoing incision and drainage, puncture, or other invasive procedures, color or power Doppler imaging is important to map out surrounding vasculature beforehand (**Fig. 4**).[7,8]

When choosing the optimal transducer, remember that higher-frequency transducers provide better spatial resolution but at the expense of lower penetration into tissues.[3] Because most musculoskeletal applications are superficial, it is appropriate to use the highest frequency transducer available. When interrogating deeper structures or in patients with abundant soft tissue overlying the target structure, a lower-frequency transducer with a broader footprint typically allows better visualization (**Figs. 5** and **6**).

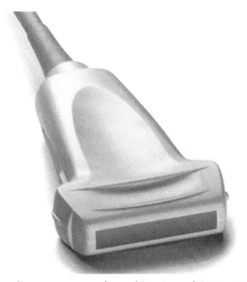

Fig. 2. High-frequency linear array transducer. (*Courtesy of* T. Wu, MD, Phoenix, AZ.)

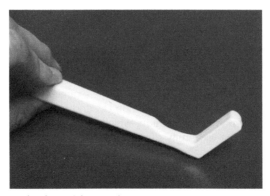

Fig. 3. High-frequency hockey stick transducer.

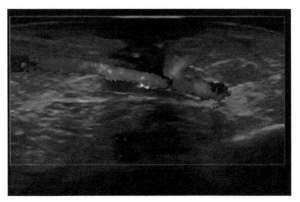

Fig. 4. US image of a skin ulcer with an underlying abscess. Note the vessel highlighted by color Doppler.

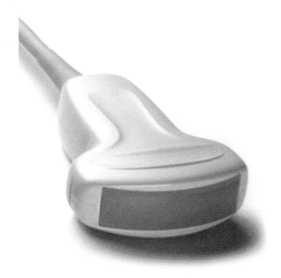

Fig. 5. Low-frequency curvilinear transducer with a large footprint. (*Courtesy of* T. Wu, MD, Phoenix, AZ.)

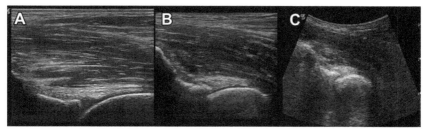

Fig. 6. Images of the right hip in a small adult woman using three different transducers: (A) obtained using a linear 14 MHz transducer, (B) obtained using a linear 6-MHz transducer, and (C) obtained using a 4-MHz curvilinear transducer. Note, that higher-frequency transducers provide better resolution and detail. The lower the frequency of the transducer, the better the visualization of deeper structures. (*Data from* Jacobson JA. Fundamentals of musculoskeletal ultrasound. Philadelphia: Saunders; 2007.)

MAXIMIZING IMAGE QUALITY

Patient and examiner comfort allow for the best images and most confident diagnosis with bedside US. Helping patients to settle into a comfortable position enhances their ability to cooperate with the scan. The sonographer should seek a relaxed hand position and grip on the probe. Resting the ulnar side of the hand on the patient and holding the transducer like a pencil allow for fine controlled movements to bring the area of interest into focus (**Fig. 7**). This also allows the examiner to use the other hand to palpate and reposition the extremity, thereby combining the physical examination with US imaging.

Using copious gel serves as an acoustic window to optimize image capture. This reduces the amount of pressure applied to obtain an adequate image. A water bath can optimize inspection of very superficial abnormalities and eliminate contact over painful areas being examined (**Figs. 8** and **9**). This technique is useful on digits, hands, and feet and in small children.[9] Some sonographers advocate use of US standoff pads; however many practitioners find these cumbersome and difficult to secure into place.

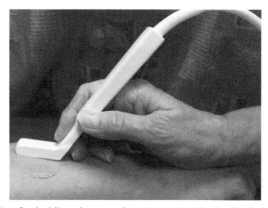

Fig. 7. Hand position for holding the transducer in a grip identical to holding a pencil. Note the base of the sonographer's hand rests on the model's arm. This allows maximal control for fine motions.

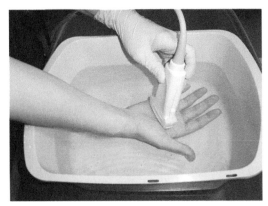

Fig. 8. Water immersion technique to create an acoustic window. (*Courtesy of* T. Wu, MD, Phoenix, AZ.)

At the beginning of the examination, evaluate surrounding normal tissue first. Then, gently slide the transducer toward the affected area, noting changes in the US appearance of underlying structures (**Fig. 10**). The patient can help guide to the most symptomatic area. As with most imaging modalities, obtain multiple views of the symptomatic area in different planes. Transducer compression adds dynamic information, as does having the patient move the extremity during the scan. Capture both still images and video/cine clips for subsequent review.[3]

In many musculoskeletal scans, the area of interest is too large to capture on one image alone. If unable to visualize the entire structure in one view, use an extended view with dual-screen images to capture the scope of the abnormality (**Figs. 11** and **12**). Dual-screen capability also allows side-by-side comparison of normal and abnormal structures.[10] It is often useful to capture an image of the unaffected contralateral side for comparison. Some US units have extended field of view or panoramic capability, which can lengthen the field of view to 10 or 15 cm.

NORMAL STRUCTURES
Skin

Dermis and epidermis appear as a thin, linear echogenic stripe on US. In standard clinical settings, the two layers cannot be distinguished by US (**Fig. 13**).[11]

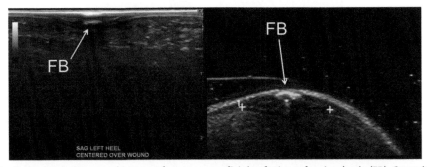

Fig. 9. Sagittal ultrasound image of a very superficial soft tissue foreign body (FB). Scanning with gel alone makes it difficult to visualize the FB (*left*). Immersing the extremity into a water bath brings the FB into focus (*right*).

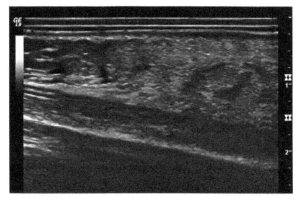

Fig. 10. Longitudinal image of subcutaneous soft tissue demonstrating transition from normal tissue on the left, into a region affected by cellulitis on the right.

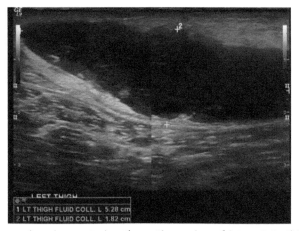

Fig. 11. Dual-screen imaging capturing the entire region of interest. In this example, the large fluid collection in a patient's thigh can be optimally delineated.

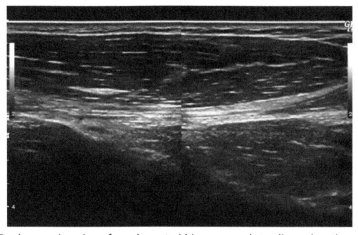

Fig. 12. Dual-screen imaging of an elongated biceps musculotendinous junction.

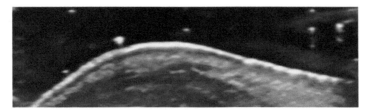

Fig. 13. Magnified image of subcutaneous tissues of a finger demonstrating dermis/epidermis as a smooth curvilinear echogenic stripe overlying the other tissues. Note that copious gel on the extremity (overlying hypoechoic layer) allows better visualization of very superficial structures.

Subcutaneous Fat

Normal adipose tissue appears hypoechoic with thin, linear echogenic septations separating fat lobules. The septations generally run parallel to the overlying skin surface (**Figs. 14** and **15**).

Muscle

The morphology of normal muscle tissue is clearly evident on US. Multiple muscle fascicles are bundled together to form a muscle belly. A sheath called the perimysium surrounds the entire structure. Muscle fascicles appear relatively hypoechoic compared with the hyperechoic encasing linear septations and sheath (**Fig. 16**). On short-axis images, muscle septations appear as white dots on a hypoechoic background.[3]

Lymph Nodes

Normal lymph nodes typically appear kidney bean or dumbbell shaped. The hypoechoic cortex wraps around the inner fatty (hyperechoic) hilum. Normal vascularity enters at the hilum and branches into the central portion of the node (**Fig. 17**).[12]

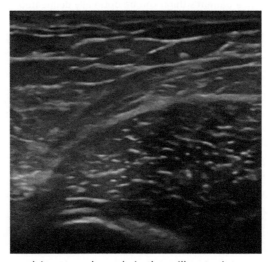

Fig. 14. Fat lobules overlying normal muscle in the axillary region.

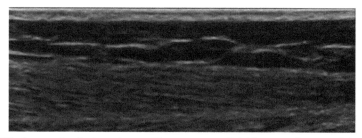

Fig. 15. US of normal soft tissue layers. The most superficial layer at the top of the screen is the dermis/epidermis. The next layer consists of hypoechoic fat lobules, separated by linear echogenic striations. The deepest layer is muscle tissue, which may appear relatively hyperechoic or isoechoic to normal adipose tissue.

Bone

The surface of bone reflects US, appearing as an echogenic linear structure parallel to the skin surface. The US beam is completely reflected by cortex, which produces shadowing posteriorly. When bone is insonated with a perpendicular sound beam, reverberation can occur (**Fig. 18**).[13]

Joints

Most joints may be segmentally visualized by US (**Fig. 19**). Joints are large complex structures, and only a small portion can be visualized at any time with 2-D US. Cartilage lining an articular surface appears as a smooth, anechoic layer. Joints are surrounded by ligaments and tendons and contain additional cushioning structures, such as labra and menisci, a portion of which can be studied with bedside sonography. Normal joints contain a small amount of fluid, which can be seen as an anechoic or hypoechoic collection in between the bony surfaces (**Fig. 20**).

Tendons

Normal tendon has a characteristic US appearance. A bandlike structure with parallel alternating hyperechoic and hypoechoic linear striations is identified on long-axis imaging (**Fig. 21**). On short-axis images, tendons appear oval shaped and contain multiple dots (**Fig. 22**).[14,15] Normal tendons demonstrate no vascularity on color flow imaging.

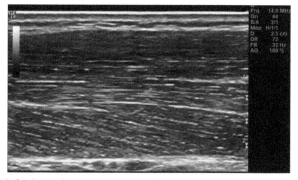

Fig. 16. Long-axis high-resolution US image of a normal gastrocnemius muscle.

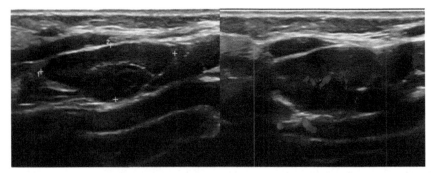

Fig. 17. US of a normal lymph node on B-mode scanning (*left*) and with color Doppler (*right*).

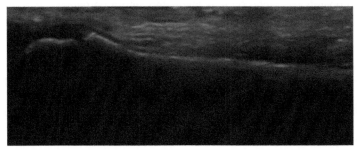

Fig. 18. High-frequency linear US image of a metacarpal. The cortex appears as a smooth echogenic line, with posterior shadowing.

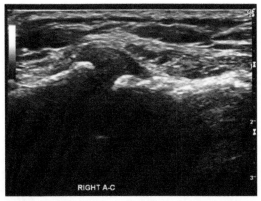

Fig. 19. Long-axis view of a right acromioclavicular joint showing the distal tip of the clavicle at its articulation with the acromion.

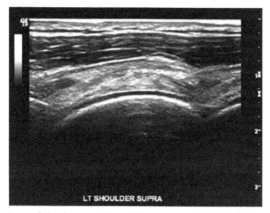

Fig. 20. Short-axis view of the humeral head shows a smooth curvilinear anechoic rim outlining the bony cortex. This layer correlates with articular cartilage and should not be confused with fluid in the joint.

The musculotendinous junction of tendons can be identified by tracing back from the tendinous insertion toward the muscle belly. Ligaments, which attach bone to bone, have a similar appearance, but are shorter and more compact (**Fig. 23**).[14]

ARTIFACTS

Artifacts important in musculoskeletal sonography are consistent with those encountered in all other US imaging. One artifact that is uniquely important for imaging of tendons, however, is seldom an issue in other body parts. This artifact is called anisotropy and is related to the angle of the incident US beam.

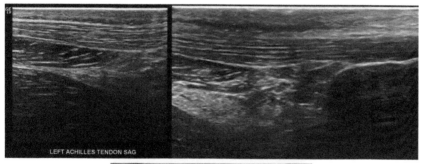

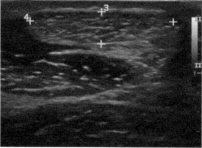

Fig. 21. Long-axis and short-axis US images of an Achilles tendon. The classic fibrillar pattern is evident on the longitudinal view.

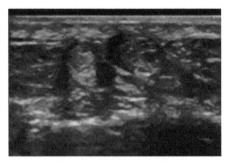

Fig. 22. Short-axis US image of the flexor tendons on the palmar aspect of the hand. Note each rounded tendon demonstrates the classic pattern of tiny dots on a hypoechoic background.

When an ultrasound wave strikes the surface of a structure at a perpendicular angle, the normal tendon fibrillar pattern is well delineated. When the angle is not perpendicular, however, this pattern is lost, and the tendon demonstrates areas of hypoechogenicity (**Fig. 24**). This may be confused with tendon injury.[16]

SONOGRAPHIC APPEARANCES OF MUSCULOSKELETAL PATHOLOGY
Cellulitis

US appearance of cellulitis depends on severity and stage of infection. Initial findings are of overall thickening of the subcutaneous soft tissue, loss of normal architecture, and diffuse increase in echogenicity of skin and underlying adipose (**Fig. 25**). The linear septations that separate fat lobules become indistinct. This classic appearance of cellulitis is typically visualized within the first few days of the infection.[17]

The thickening and increased echogenicity of cellulitis seen on US is nonspecific and can be seen in other entities causing soft tissue edema. As infection progresses, particularly without treatment, fluid channels may appear, separating the inflamed hyperechoic fat lobules (**Fig. 26**).[18]

As infection progresses, more severe edema manifests as prominent, linear, or branching hypoechoic or anechoic areas of fluid within the interlobular septae, interspersed with hyperechoic inflamed fat globules (**Fig. 27**). The appearance is termed cobblestoning.[19]

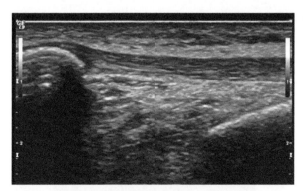

Fig. 23. Longitudinal gray-scale image demonstrating the upper segment of the patellar "tendon." The bandlike structure attaching the inferior margin of the patella to the tibial tuberosity is actually a ligament but is referred to as a tendon in clinical practice.

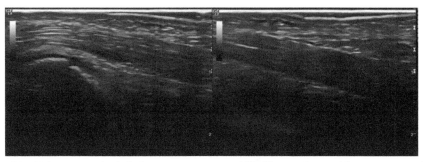

Fig. 24. US image on the left demonstrates normal fibrillar tendon architecture. Note this normal pattern is best identified as the tendon drapes over the humeral head (*left side*). Image on right shows signal dropout within the tendon as the transducer angle moves away from perpendicular. This is due to anisotropy artifact.

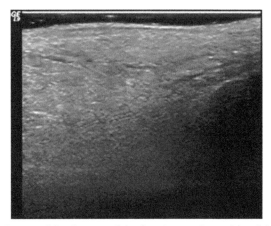

Fig. 25. Gray-scale image of the dorsum of the foot in a patient with mild cellulitis. Note loss of distinct fat lobules, and the uniform hyperechoic appearance of subcutaneous adipose tissue.

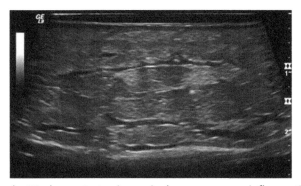

Fig. 26. Gray-scale US demonstrates increasingly more severe inflammation. Branching linear fluid collections are seen interspersed among the hyperechoic fat lobules.

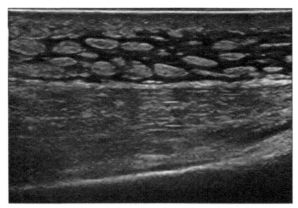

Fig. 27. Severe extensive cellulitis, manifesting on US as a cobblestone appearance, over the healthy underlying muscle tissue.

Phlegmon

As an area of cellulitis becomes more organized, it forms a phlegmon. The typical appearance of a phlegmon on US is a poorly circumscribed, hypoechoic area, with ill-defined borders (**Fig. 28**). Gentle ballottement over the area with an US probe may cause the phlegmon to dissipate into the surrounding tissue.

Abscess

Mature soft-tissue abscesses appear as distinct hypoechoic fluid collections on US. Occasionally, an abscess is hyperechoic to adjacent tissues. Heterogeneous components, debris, and septations are not uncommon (**Fig. 29**).[19]

It is sometimes difficult to distinguish a drainable abscess from a phlegmon. Abscesses typically demonstrate posterior acoustic enhancement on US, but this is not always the case. Gentle ballottement over an abscess should not dissipate its contents and instead produces a swirling motion of internal fluid. Color flow or power Doppler may show hyperemia in the rim of surrounding tissue. On occasion, a soft tissue abscess may contain air, which manifests as punctate echogenic foci and associated ringdown artifact on US (**Fig. 30**).

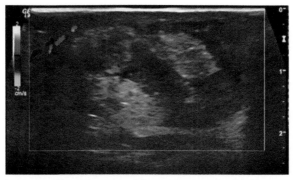

Fig. 28. Gray-scale image of a phlegmon with superimposed color flow. Note the extensive inflammation of subcutaneous tissue without a distinct fluid collection.

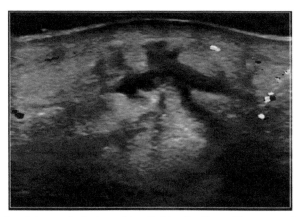

Fig. 29. US of a focal, hypoechoic, branching fluid collection with surrounding cellulitis and hyperemia within the soft tissue. These findings are consistent with a subcutaneous abscess.

Lymphadenitis

Reactive lymph nodes in the region of infection or inflammation typically enlarge in size, however, maintain their normal shape and architecture. Overall length is less important than the width, which should not exceed 1 cm in benign processes.[12] On US, a normal lymph node should have a kidney bean shape, with symmetric cortical thickness, echogenic fatty hilum, and centrally located vasculature (**Fig. 31**).

As inflammation progresses, lymph nodes can become necrotic. A necrotic lymph node loses its kidney bean shape and appears more oval on US. Distinction between the cortex and hilum may be lost and hyperemia is evident throughout the structure. If an abscess forms, focal areas of central liquefaction become evident (**Fig. 32**). A rounded lymph node should raise suspicion for malignancy (**Fig. 33**).

Myositis

Muscle tissue inflammation can occur secondary to infection, trauma, vasculitis, or autoimmune disease. In early stages of myositis, the muscle belly becomes

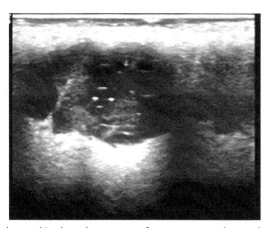

Fig. 30. An abscess located in the subcutaneous fat appears as a hypoechoic lesion with posterior acoustic enhancement. Note scattered debris and punctate hyperechoic foci, representative of internal air bubbles.

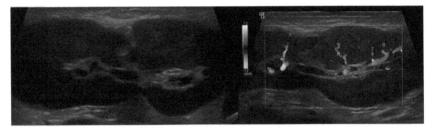

Fig. 31. Large inguinal lymph node in B-mode (*left*) and with color flow applied (*right*). Although this node is large, normal architecture is maintained, including its dumbbell shape, gently lobular contour, hypoechoic cortex, hyperechoic fatty hilum, and central vascularity.

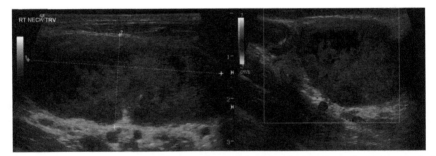

Fig. 32. Gray-scale (*left*) and color flow US images (*right*) of a lymph node with central abscess formation. The structure is no longer dumbbell shaped, and size is increased. Distinction between the hilum and cortex is lost, and there is central hypoechoic liquefaction.

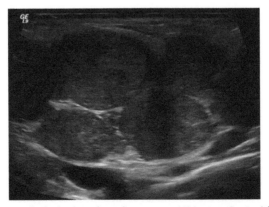

Fig. 33. Rounded supraclavicular lymph nodes seen on US in a patient with lymphoma. Note the loss of the central fatty hila.

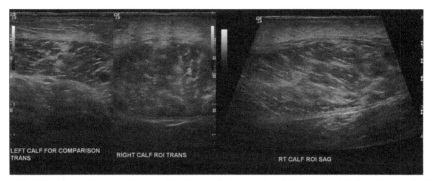

LEFT CALF FOR COMPARISON TRANS   RIGHT CALF ROI TRANS   RT CALF ROI SAG

Fig. 34. US of a patient with myositis. The left image is of his normal left calf muscle for comparison. Short-axis (*middle image*) and long-axis (*right image*) views of the inflamed muscle demonstrate enlargement of the muscle belly with distortion of the interfascicular septations.

edematous, resulting in diffuse enlargement and relative increase in overall echogenicity (**Fig. 34**). These alterations are best appreciated by comparison with adjacent or contralateral muscle groups. If necrosis occurs, hyperechoic foci or a frank abscess may be visible on US.[20]

Pyomyositis is a muscle infection commonly associated with abscess formation. It is most frequently seen in immunocompromised patients and in the large muscles of the lower extremities. Overlying skin and subcutaneous tissues are either mildly involved or not involved at all. Early inflammatory changes demonstrate echogenic septae within the muscle, sometimes visible along fascial planes. A phlegmon can develop in the early stages and lead to liquefaction and abscess formation if left untreated. On US, hypoechoic fluid collections can be seen within the muscle belly and fibrous septae (**Figs. 35** and **36**). Increased color flow within the region may also be noted at the bedside.[18,19]

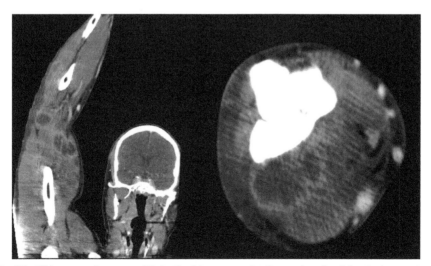

Fig. 35. CT images of pyomyositis in the biceps muscle. Coronal and axial cuts demonstrate multifocal hypoattenuating, rim-enhancing areas within the muscle throughout the arm.

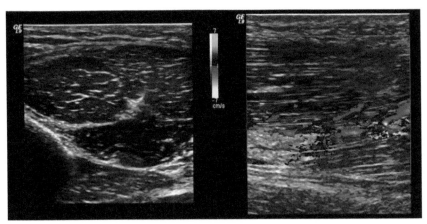

Fig. 36. US images of the same patient with pyomyositis from **Fig. 35** demonstrating hypo-echoic fluid collections within the biceps muscle belly (*left image*) and hyperemia on color flow evaluation of the muscle (*right image*).

Soft Tissue Hematoma

The extremely variable US appearances of subcutaneous hematomas can generate confusion in some clinical settings. A history of trauma may not always be recalled. These fluid collections are typically oval or round, and may have lobular contours. The fibrous capsule, which develops around hematomas, gives these lesions a sharply circumscribed margin. In the acute phase (days to weeks), the fluid collection is more hypoechoic (**Fig. 37**). As the hematoma ages (weeks to months), it can appear more hyperechoic and blend into the surrounding tissue on US. Mural nodules or internal septations can develop in later stages (**Fig. 38**).

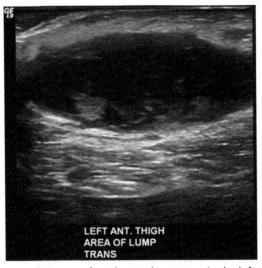

Fig. 37. Long-axis gray-scale image of a subacute hematoma in the left thigh. The crescent-shaped, hypoechoic fluid collection contains internal debris.

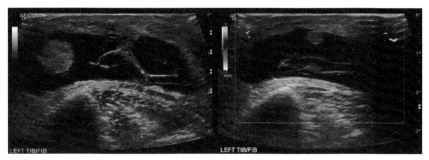

Fig. 38. Gray-scale (*left image*) and color flow (*right image*) US of a resolving hematoma in the left calf. This collection demonstrates irregular septations and nodular components, which are avascular. Evolving blood collections tend to develop fibrin strands after 1–2 weeks.

If a hematoma is suspected on US, clinical correlation is usually required. Diagnostic accuracy can be improved by performing serial US examinations and monitoring resolution and reabsorption of the hematoma over time.[21]

Soft Tissue Foreign Bodies

US is ideal for imaging foreign bodies within the soft tissues. Conventionally, radiography was used to search for foreign material; however, many foreign bodies are not visible on standard radiographs. Wooden foreign material; plant material, such as thorns; and some glass foreign bodies are not opaque on radiographs. On US, all types of foreign bodies appear hyperechoic (**Figs. 39** and **40**). Many foreign bodies have a surrounding hypoechoic halo of edema and tissue reaction. With small foreign bodies, look for other US findings, such as shadowing, reverberation artifact, distortion of normal tissue architecture, and surrounding hyperemia with color flow imaging.[20,22]

Soft tissue gas can be a confounding factor when looking for a foreign body on US. Air bubbles cause shadowing and occasionally reverberation artifacts on US (**Fig. 41**). It is often difficult to determine if there is a foreign body present when there is air in the region of interest.

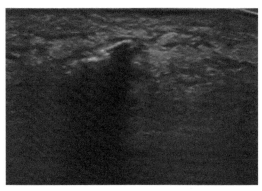

Fig. 39. US of a hyperechoic foreign body in the soft tissue. Note the shadow posterior to the foreign body.

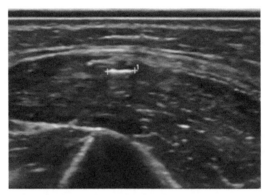

Fig. 40. US of small foreign body overlying the distal humerus. Small foreign bodies (<3 mm) may not produce acoustic shadowing.

Muscle Injuries

US can detect muscle injuries, such as contusions, strains, tears, or lacerations. The severity of injury can be graded by the following criteria:

Grade 1: No significant fiber disruption
Grade 2: Moderate disruption
Grade 3: Complete fiber disruption

A muscle contusion appears on US as a focal or widespread area of decreased echogenicity, with loss of the normal, feathery pattern of muscle fascicles (**Fig. 42**). Acute contusions are seen as blood dissecting between the fascicles. Within 3 or 4 days, the margins of the contusion typically become more defined and a focal hematoma may be noted.

Muscle strains and tears can also be detected via bedside US. The most common sites of injury are along the myotendinous junction and the peripheral area of the muscle belly that is covered by perimysium (**Fig. 43**).[23–25]

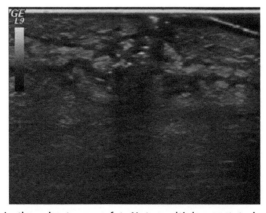

Fig. 41. US of air in the subcutaneous fat. Note multiple punctate hyperechoic foci and irregular areas of dirty shadowing.

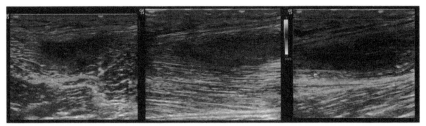

Fig. 42. US images of a muscle contusion. Short-axis view (*left*), long-axis view (*middle*), and color flow imaging (*right*) demonstrating hypoechoic fluid collections in the muscle belly with loss of normal muscle architecture in the area of the contusion.

Joint Effusions

US has been used for more than two decades in diagnosing joint effusions and guiding arthrocenteses in pediatric hips. It can also be used at the bedside in adults to determine if an effusion is present, and to guide arthrocentesis and joint injection attempts.[26,27] A joint effusion appears as a hypoechoic collection between the articular surfaces (**Figs. 44** and **45**). During US-guided joint aspiration or injection, the needle can be visualized entering the joint space, thereby minimizing the number of attempts required for successful aspiration or injection.

Popliteal Cysts

Normal bursae around joints are not visible by US unless distended by fluid. Knee effusions may extend into the popliteal fossa through a bursa between the medial head of the gastrocnemius and the semimembranosus tendon. This collection of fluid is commonly called a Baker or popliteal cyst. Baker cysts produce a beaklike collection

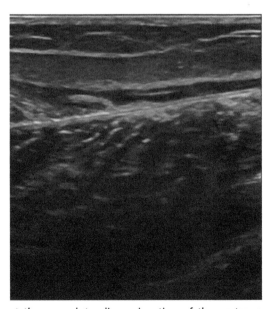

Fig. 43. Focal tear at the musculotendinous junction of the gastrocnemius presents as a linear fluid collection and retraction of muscle fibers along the central tendon.

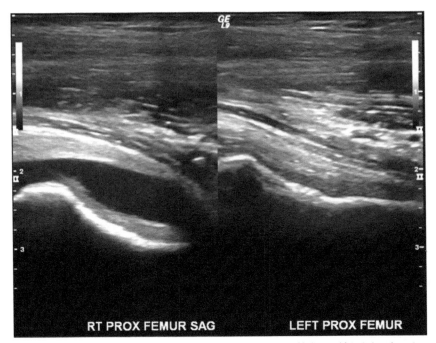

Fig. 44. Dual-screen US image demonstrating long-axis views of bilateral hip joints in a 4-year-old boy presenting with a limp. On the image on the left, a crescent-shaped, hypoechoic effusion is identified in the right hip joint in this child with septic arthritis. Compare to the image on the right, which demonstrates the normal appearance of the child's contralateral hip.

of fluid on bedside US (**Fig. 46**).[28] When patients have a ruptured Baker cyst, a bedside US demonstrates irregular collections of hypoechoic or anechoic fluid around the inferior margin of the bursa. Fluid may track inferiorly down the calf around the medial head of the gastrocnemius (**Fig. 47**).

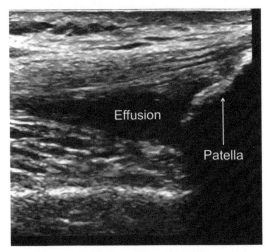

Fig. 45. Long-axis view of the suprapatellar region of a left knee demonstrating a joint effusion below the fibrillated appearance of the quadriceps tendon as it inserts into the patella.

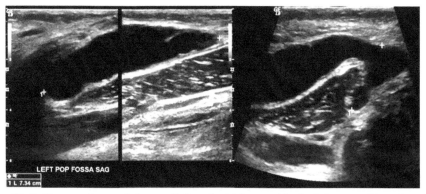

Fig. 46. Split screen long axis image (*left and middle panels*) of a Baker cyst. Note that the fluid collection within the popliteal fossa has a beaklike appearance extending along the medial head of the gastrocnemius (*right panel*).

Fractures

Because normal bones have a smooth linear surface, fractures can be easily detected on US by looking for a breach in the cortex (**Fig. 48**). The sensitivity of US in diagnosing rib and sternal fractures exceeds that of radiographs.[13,26,29] US can distinguish between a simple cortical buckle and a displaced fracture; however, accurately documenting angulation, distraction or displacement is beyond the scope of this modality.

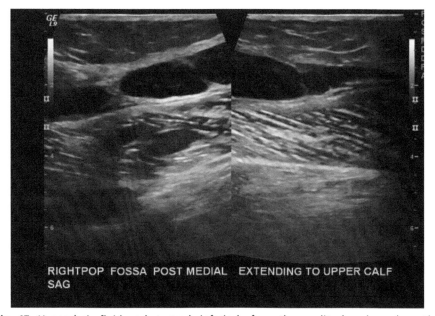

Fig. 47. Hypoechoic fluid pockets track inferiorly from the popliteal region, along the medial head of the gastrocnemius muscle from a ruptured Baker cyst, as demonstrated on this dual screen ultrasound image.

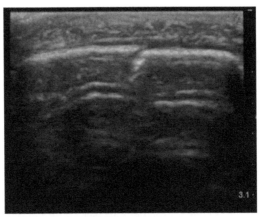

Fig. 48. US of a patellar fracture. The smooth hyperechoic linear cortex is interrupted by a fracture line. (*Courtesy of* T. Wu, MD, Phoenix, AZ.)

Periostitis

Periosteal reactions may be seen in healing fractures, infection, or other bony destructive processes. US is more sensitive than other imaging modalities for detecting subtle periostitis (**Fig. 49**).[13,27]

Osteomyelitis

Studies have shown that osteomyelitis may manifest as visible elevated periosteum on US, with associated edema or abscess (**Figs. 50 and 51**).[13,27]

Tendon Injuries

Tendons have a uniform appearance throughout the body. On US, normal tendons have uniform thickness with typical fibrillar pattern seen on long-axis views (**Fig. 52**).[14] Tendonitis can be seen on US as thickening of the fibers and loss of the

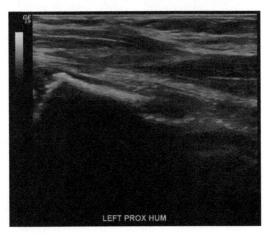

Fig. 49. The linear cortex of the proximal humerus in this 4-year-old girl is interrupted by a focus of periosteal infection. This abnormality was not detected on plain radiographs, and was less conspicuous on the MRI than it was on the US.

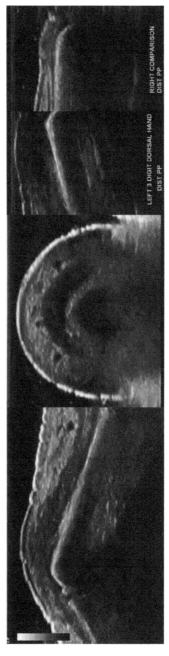

Fig. 50. US images of the third finger in an 8 year-old boy with a periosteal abscess. Long-axis view (*left*), short-axis view (*middle*), and comparison views of the contralateral side (*right*) demonstrate periosteal reaction and a hypoechoic fluid collection along the bony cortex.

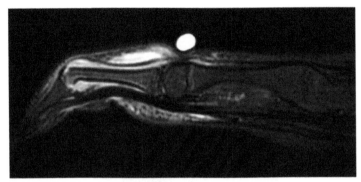

Fig. 51. MRI with T2-weighted imaging of the same patient in **Fig. 50** showing a rim of high signal fluid surrounding the affected digit.

normal fibrillar echotexture. As inflammation progresses, there is displacement of the normal fibers of the tendon with areas of hypoechogenicity. Power Doppler can be applied to the relaxed tendon to look for neovascularity, when chronic tendonitis is suspected (**Fig. 53**).

Inflammation can involve the synovial sheath surrounding many tendons. This condition, known as tenosynovitis, can be detected on bedside US. With tenosynovitis, fluid is visualized surrounding an otherwise normal appearing tendon (**Fig. 54**).[14]

In addition to tendon inflammation, acute tendon injuries are easily detected via bedside US. When a tendon is ruptured or injured, a hypoechoic defect is seen within the tendon fibers on US.[30,31] With a full tendon rupture, it is also possible to visualize the torn end of the tendon retracted proximal to the normal insertion site (**Fig. 55**).

Joint Prostheses

Recent studies on the use of US in the evaluation of joint prostheses show that bedside US is capable of detecting fluid collections and joint effusions surrounding implanted hardware (**Fig. 56**).[32]

Sebaceous Cysts

Also known as epidermal inclusion cysts, sebaceous cysts are epithelial-lined structures filled with keratin and other debris. On US, sebaceous cysts appear as

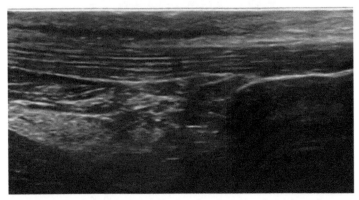

Fig. 52. Long-axis view of a normal Achilles tendon insertion into the calcaneus. Note the fibrillar appearance of the tendon.

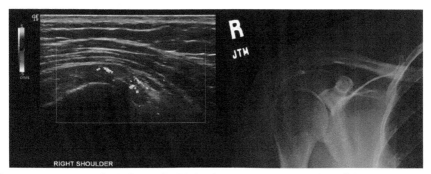

Fig. 53. A US image of calcific tendonitis in the supraspinatus tendon of the right shoulder (*left image*). Note the foci of increased color flow superimposed on areas of decreased echogenicity. On the patient's radiograph (*right image*), a focus of mineralization in the supraspinatus tendon can be seen.

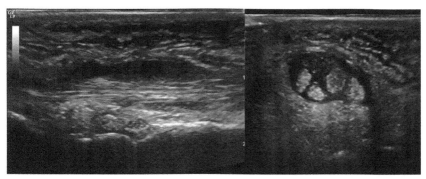

Fig. 54. Long-axis (*left*) and short-axis (*right*) views of the extensor tendons on the dorsum of the hand in a patient with tenosynovitis. Note the normal tendon fibrillar pattern is maintained but there is fluid surrounding the tendons.

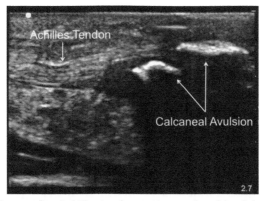

Fig. 55. Long-axis image of an Achilles tendon rupture and avulsion injury of the calcaneus. Note the wavy appearance of the retracted and torn tendon. (*Courtesy of* T. Wu, MD, Phoenix, AZ.)

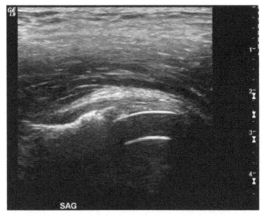

Fig. 56. Long-axis US image of a right hip total arthroplasty. The bony acetabulum and intact polyethylene liner (*two parallel hyperechoic lines*) can be identified. Overlying muscles appear intact. No fluid is identified in this asymptomatic hip.

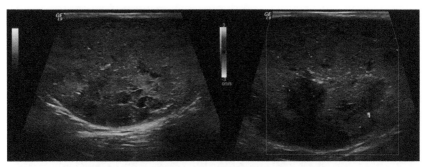

Fig. 57. Gray-scale (*left*) and color flow (*right*) images of a sebaceous cyst. This well-circumscribed oval-shaped lesion demonstrates heterogeneous content, posterior acoustic enhancement, and no internal color flow.

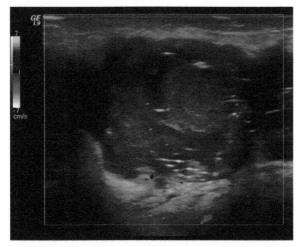

Fig. 58. Gray-scale with color imaging of a pilonidal cyst overlying the sacrococcygeal region. The linear areas of echogenicity represent hairs within the pilonidal cyst.

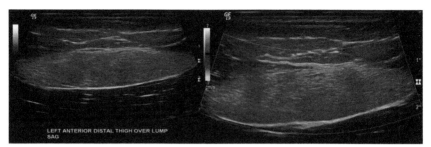

Fig. 59. Gray-scale (*left image*) and color flow (*right image*) scans of a benign soft tissue lipoma. Lipomas can demonstrate any echogenicity in relation to surrounding tissue.

superficial, circumscribed, round, or oval masses with internal heterogeneous architecture. Color flow should not be detected within the cyst (**Fig. 57**). Occasionally, a sebaceous cyst shows a focal dermal attachment and/or a concentric ring or target pattern. When a sebaceous cyst ruptures, it demonstrates a lobulated or lopsided shape on bedside US. There may be an increase in surrounding inflammatory soft tissue reaction on color Doppler.[33,34]

Pilonidal Cysts

A common condition overlying the sacrococcygeal region, these pseudocystic lesions (pilonidal cysts) tend to appear as an oval or round complex fluid collection with mixed echogenicity on bedside US. Linear hypoechoic structures within the cyst correspond to internal hairs (**Fig. 58**). Posterior acoustic enhancement may be seen and increased vascularity in the surrounding tissue may be visualized with color imaging.[33] Bedside US is useful in delineating the extent of the cyst and the best tract for incision and drainage.

Lipomas

Lipomas, common soft tissue lesions, may demonstrate any echogenicity. They may be difficult to detect on US because they can blend into the surrounding adipose tissue. When seen, color flow imaging should not show any internal vascularity (**Fig. 59**). The best use of US in evaluating lipomas is its use to distinguish between a benign lipoma and more ominous solid lesions.[35]

SUMMARY

Used as an extension of the physical examination, point-of-care bedside US can help facilitate diagnoses and aide in structuring management of many patients with musculoskeletal complaints and soft tissue abnormalities. US is often better than plain radiographs, CT, and MRI in evaluating some musculoskeletal complaints and is especially useful in assessing patients too unstable for transport or who are situated in resource-limited environments. The use of musculoskeletal ultrasonography will continue to evolve along with the technologic advances that lend to its utility at the bedside.

REFERENCES

1. Kane D, Grassi W, Sturrock R, et al. A brief history of musculoskeletal ultrasound: "from bats and ships to babies and hips". Rheumatology 2004;43:931–3.

2. Hwang JQ, Kimberly HH, Liteplo AS, et al. An evidence-based approach to emergency ultrasound. Emerg Med Pract 2011;13(3):1–27.
3. Jacobson JA. Fundamentals of musculoskeletal ultrasound. Philadelphia: Saunders; 2007.
4. Jamadar DA, Jacobson JA, Caoili EM, et al. Musculoskeletal sonography technique: focused versus comprehensive evaluation. AJR Am J Roentgenol 2008; 190:5–9.
5. Nazarian I. The top 10 reasons musculoskeletal sonography is an important complementary or alternative technique to MRI. AJR Am J Roentgenol 2008;190: 1621–6.
6. Khoury V, Cardinal E, Bureau NJ. Musculoskeletal sonography: a dynamic tool for usual and unusual disorders. AJR Am J Roentgenol 2007;188:W63–73.
7. Newman JS, Adler RS, Bude RO, et al. Detection of soft tissue hyperemia: value of power doppler sonography. AJR Am J Roentgenol 1994;163:385–9.
8. Blaivas M, Srikar A. Unexpected findings on point of care superficial ultrasound imaging before incision and drainage. J Ultrasound Med 2011;30:1425–30.
9. Blaivas M, Lyon M, Brannam L, et al. Water bath evaluation technique for emergency ultrasound of painful superficial structures. Am J Emerg Med 2004;22: 589–93.
10. Lin EC, Middleton WD, Teefey SA. Extended field-of-view sonography in musculoskeletal imaging. J Ultrasound Med 1991;18(2):156–67.
11. Worstman X. Common applications of dermatologic sonography. J Ultrasound Med 2012;31:97–111.
12. Whitman GJ, Lu TJ, Adejolu M, et al. Lymph node sonography. Ultrasound Clin 2011;6:369–80.
13. Cho KH, Lee YH, Lee SM, et al. Sonography of bone and bone-related diseases of the extremities. J Clin Ultrasound 2004;32:511–21.
14. Dillehay GL, Deschler T, Rogers LF, et al. The ultrasonographic characterization of tendons. Invest Radiol 1984;19:338–41.
15. Carr JC, Hanly S, Griffin J, et al. Sonography of the patellar tendon and adjacent structures in pediatric and adult patients. AJR Am J Roentgenol 2001;176: 1535–9.
16. Scanlan KA. Sonographic artifacts and their origins. AJR Am J Roentgenol 1991; 156:1267.
17. Loyer EM, DuBrow RA, David CL, et al. Imaging of superficial soft-tissue infection: sonographic findings in cases of cellulitis and abscess. AJR Am J Roentgenol 1996;166:149–52.
18. Bureau NJ, Chem RK, Cardinal E. Musculoskeletal infections: US manifestations. Radiographics 1999;19:1585–92.
19. Chau CL, Griffith JF. Musculoskeletal infections: ultrasound appearances. Clin Radiol 2005;60:149–59.
20. Horton LK, Jacobson JA, Powell A, et al. Sonography and radiography of soft-tissue foreign bodies. AJR Am J Roentgenol 2001;176:1155–9.
21. Wu S, Tu R, Liu G, et al. Role of ultrasound in the diagnosis of common soft tissue lesions of the limbs. Ultrasound Q 2013;29(1):67–71.
22. Boyse T, Fessell D, Jacobson J, et al. US of soft tissue foreign bodies and associated complications with surgical correlation. Radiographics 2001;21:1251–6.
23. Lee JC, Healy JC. Sonography of lower limb muscle injury. AJR Am J Roentgenol 2004;182:341–51.
24. Jamadar DA, Jacobson JA, Theisen SE, et al. Sonography of the painful calf: differential considerations. AJR Am J Roentgenol 2002;179:709–16.

25. Fessell DP, Jacobson JA, Craig J, et al. Using sonography to reveal and aspirate joint effusions. AJR Am J Roentgenol 2000;174:1353–62.
26. Turk F, Kurt AB, Saglam S, et al. Evaluation by ultrasound of traumatic rib fractures missed by radiography. Emerg Radiol 2010;17:473–7.
27. Wenaden AE, Szyszko TA, Saifuddin A. Imaging of periosteal reactions associated with focal lesions of bone. Clin Radiol 2005;60:439–56.
28. Constantino DG, Roemer B, Leber EH. Septic arthritis and bursitis: emergency ultrasound can facilitate diagnosis. J Emerg Med 2007;32:295–7.
29. Wood J, Dal MY. Diagnostic value of sonographic assessment of sternal fractures compared with conventional radiography and bone scans. J Ultrasound Med 2006;25:1263–8.
30. Wu TS, Roque PJ, Green J, et al. Bedside ultrasound evaluation of tendon injuries. Am J Emerg Med 2012;30:1617–21.
31. Robinson P. Sonography of common tendon injuries. AJR Am J Roentgenol 2009; 193:607–18.
32. Long S, Surrey D, Nazarian L. Common sonographic findings in the painful hip after arthroplasty. J Ultrasound Med 2012;31:301–12.
33. Hwang S. Sonographic evaluation of musculoskeletal soft tissue masses. Ultrasound Q 2005;21:259–70.
34. Huang C, Sheung-Fat K, Hsuan-Ying H, et al. Epidermal cysts in the superficial soft tissues. J Ultrasound Med 2011;30:111–7.
35. Crundwell N, O'Donnell A, Saifuddin A. Non-neoplastic conditions presenting as soft tissue tumours. Clin Radiol 2007;62:18–27.

Basic Ultrasound-guided Procedures

Laurel Barr, MD[a],*, Nicholas Hatch, MD[a], Pedro J. Roque, MD[a],
Teresa S. Wu, MD[b]

KEYWORDS

- Ultrasound • Peripheral intravenous access • Central venous access
- Arterial access • Suprapubic aspiration • Abscess incision and drainage
- Foreign body localization • Arthrocentesis

KEY POINTS

- Ultrasound guidance for basic procedures helps to visualize the target and surrounding structures, which saves time, increases safety, and increases first-attempt success.
- Visualizing the needle in long-axis views ensures that the tip of the needle remains in the target structure.
- Color flow or Doppler can be used to help identify a target vessel as an artery or a vein.
- Ultrasound can detect radiolucent foreign bodies such as plastic or wood.
- When using ultrasound to evaluate painful joints, use the contralateral joint for comparison.

INTRODUCTION

The use of ultrasound guidance for bedside procedures is gaining popularity in multiple clinical settings. Using ultrasound during standard procedures has been shown to increase patient safety, save time, and improve chances of success. This article discusses ultrasound guidance for basic procedures performed at the bedside. It reviews the indications and complications of the procedure, advantages of ultrasound guidance, important anatomy and sonographic correlation, and procedural technique.

Ultrasound-guided Procedures: Axis and Orientation

When performing an ultrasound-guided procedure, it is important to understand the axis and orientation of the anatomic structures and the corresponding ultrasound images produced. Vessels and other elongated structures can be visualized in the long

The authors have no disclosures or conflicts of interest.
[a] Emergency Medicine Residency, Department of Emergency Medicine, Maricopa Medical Center, 2601 East Roosevelt Street, Phoenix, AZ 85008, USA; [b] EM Residency Program, Department of Emergency Medicine, Maricopa Medical Center, School of Medicine-Phoenix, University of Arizona, 550 E Van Buren Street, Phoenix, AZ 85004, USA
* Corresponding author.
E-mail address: laurel.barr@mihs.org

Crit Care Clin 30 (2014) 275–304
http://dx.doi.org/10.1016/j.ccc.2013.10.004
0749-0704/14/$ – see front matter © 2014 Elsevier Inc. All rights reserved.

criticalcare.theclinics.com

axis or the short axis. In the short-axis view (**Fig. 1**), the ultrasound transducer is placed transverse and perpendicular to the course of the vessel, and the vessel appears as circular areas of anechoic blood. In the long-axis view (**Fig. 2**), the ultrasound transducer is placed along the course of the vessel, which produces an elongated, hypoechoic structure on two-dimensional ultrasound.

Ultrasound probes have an indicator marker on the side of the transducer. This indicator marker is typically a dot, light, or a raised line, and corresponds with the orientation marker on the ultrasound screen. By convention, during most ultrasound-guided procedures, this indicator marker should be directed toward the patient's right side for a short-axis view, or toward the patient's head for a long-axis view. The corresponding orientation marker on the ultrasound machine should be set to the upper left side of the image.

Ultrasound-guided Versus Ultrasound-assisted Procedures

Ultrasound-guided procedures are performed by visualizing the target structure with ultrasound before beginning the procedure, followed by real-time ultrasound visualization of the needle during the procedure (dynamic guidance). Ultrasound-assisted procedures are performed by visualizing the target structure with ultrasound before the procedure, and marking the site where the needle will be inserted (static guidance). The procedure is then performed without direct ultrasound visualization.[1]

Ultrasound guidance is recommended for most procedures, such as central venous access, whereas ultrasound assistance may be more useful for other procedures such as abscess incision and drainage or lumbar punctures. In many instances, the decision concerning static versus dynamic guidance depends on physician preference and clinical circumstances. If using dynamic guidance, the procedure can be performed by 1 or 2 operators using the second operator to hold the ultrasound probe while the first performs the procedure.

Ultrasound-guided Procedures: Visualizing the Needle

It is important to identify the needle and needle tip when performing an ultrasound-guided procedure. The needle appears as a brightly echogenic line or dot with an acoustic shadow and ring-down artifact farfield on the screen. Movement of the needle results in movement of the surrounding tissue, which can help to localize the needle tip.

During the initial portion of a procedure, it is often easier to attempt to visualize the needle in a short-axis view (**Fig. 3**). Once the needle trajectory is visualized, and it is

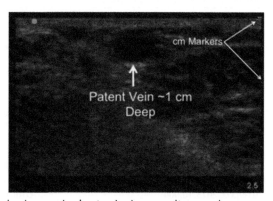

Fig. 1. A peripheral vein seen in short-axis view on ultrasound.

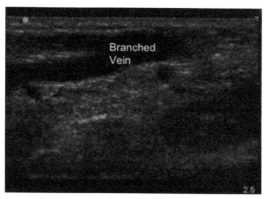

Fig. 2. A peripheral vein seen in long-axis view on ultrasound.

centered on the target structure; a long-axis approach is preferred so that the length of the needle and needle tip can be seen during the procedure (**Fig. 4**). The long-axis view allows the physician to view the needle tip at all times, and to ensure that the tip has not passed through the back of the target structure.

ULTRASOUND-GUIDED PERIPHERAL INTRAVENOUS PLACEMENT
Clinical Indications

Intravenous access is required in a variety of clinical settings. Ultrasound guidance is helpful in patients in whom intravenous (IV) access is difficult to obtain secondary to obesity, history of IV drug abuse, chemotherapy, and in those with a history of multiple IV punctures for prior treatment or evaluation. Ultrasound can also be used to access peripheral veins that are not easily palpated or have inconsistent anatomic relationships.[1] Ultrasound can locate valves and identify the presence of preexisting thrombus that may inhibit use of that particular vessel.[1,2]

Complications of any peripheral IV placement include phlebitis, infiltration, infection, artery or nerve injury, air embolism, thrombosis, hematoma, and line failure.[3,4] Real-time ultrasound guidance decreases complication rates, improves success rates, and saves time.[1,4–6] The use of ultrasound guidance for peripheral IV cannulation attempts can circumvent the need for central venous line placement or surgical cut-down to obtain IV access.[7,8]

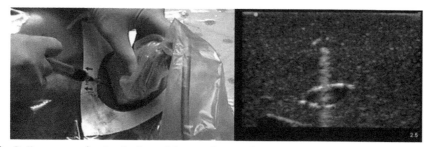

Fig. 3. Transverse, short-axis view of the needle entering a vein. Note the ring-down artifact seen on the ultrasound image farfield to the needle. The needle tip cannot be visualized, but the trajectory of the needle is clearly seen.

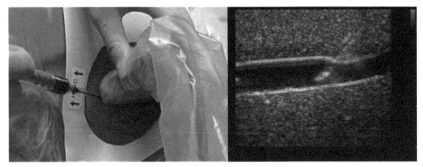

Fig. 4. Longitudinal, long-axis view of the needle entering a vein. Note that the hyperechoic needle tip is visualized puncturing the proximal vessel wall and inside the vessel lumen.

Anatomy

Ultrasound can be used to help cannulate any peripheral vein, but is typically used for access of the deep brachial vein, basilic vein, cephalic vein, and medial cubital vein. The proximal brachial vein lies in close proximity to the ulnar and median nerves, so cannulation of the more distally located deep brachial vein is preferred. The deep brachial vein is located next to the brachial artery laterally and superior to the antecubital fossa. The basilic vein is normally located radial and superficial to the brachial artery in the arm but is subject to anatomic variability.[9] The cephalic vein is deep in the radial aspect of the forearm and more superficial in the arm. The median cubital vein lies in the antecubital fossa superficial and lateral to the brachial vessels. All of these veins can easily be visualized on bedside ultrasound.

Technique

- Use a high-frequency linear array transducer to assess potential target vessels.
- Select a peripheral vein that can be easily cannulated with the highest probability of success (large superficial vein, no large valves proximal to the site of insertion, no preexisting thrombus, no overlying arteries or nerves, and no acute branches of the vessel proximal to the insertion site).
- Map out the course of the vein proximally to determine whether it courses superficially or deep.
- Apply compression with the probe to ensure that the vein collapses.
- Use color or pulsed wave Doppler to ensure that the vessel is a vein and not an artery.
- Position the patient to maximize venous pooling near the target vein.
- Place a tourniquet proximally to the target vein and prep the skin and probe in a standard fashion.
- Cover the probe with sterile plastic film if desired.
- Apply sterile ultrasound gel to the patient's skin.
- Perform the procedure using the short-axis approach (**Fig. 5**) or long-axis approach (**Fig. 6**).
- Blood will appear in the catheter reservoir once successful venous puncture has occurred.
- If the procedure is performed via the long-axis approach, ensure that the needle does not puncture the posterior wall before advancement of the IV catheter.
- Flush the catheter with normal saline and watch on ultrasound how the vein distends and bubbles are noted with saline injection.[2,3]

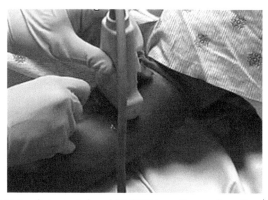

Fig. 5. Short-axis approach to peripheral IV (PIV) insertion under ultrasound guidance.

Tips

- Success with ultrasound guidance is predicted by depth and diameter of the vein. Success may be greater if the target vein is greater than 4 mm in diameter and between 3 and 15 mm deep to the skin.[10]
- For veins deeper than 1.5 cm from the surface, use a catheter that is at least 2.5 cm (2 inches) in length to prevent premature dislodgement.[10]
- Use a radial arterial line kit. These longer catheters are less prone to kinking and accidental dislodgement and the guidewire can be used to assist threading the catheter into the vessel lumen.
- Applying compression to the distal extremity causes blood to flow back into the target vein, which is called venous augmentation. Performing augmentation while visualizing Doppler flow over the target vessel can help identify the structure as a vein. Arteries continue to produce a pulsatile flow and do not show increased flow during augmentation.[11]
- Sterile technique is not required for PIV insertion, but a small sterile cover (like Tegaderm) can help minimize contamination.[3]

ULTRASOUND-GUIDED CENTRAL VENOUS ACCESS
Clinical Indications

Multiple studies have shown that the use of ultrasound increases success rates and improves patient safety during central venous access attempts. Ultrasound can be

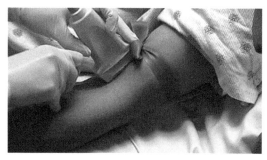

Fig. 6. Long-axis approach to PIV insertion under ultrasound guidance.

used to help guide cannulation of the internal jugular (IJ) vein, femoral veins, and subclavian veins.[1,12,13]

When performing a central venous cannulation, ultrasound guidance with direct visualization of the needle in the vein is recommended rather than ultrasound assistance. Complications of central venous cannulation include hematoma formation, air embolism, thoracic duct fistula, pneumothorax or hemothorax, venous thrombosis, infection, catheter embolism, myocardial puncture, hydromediastinum, and hydrothorax. Performing the procedure under dynamic guidance greatly reduces some of these complication rates.[1,12–15] Despite advances with ultrasound guidance, accidental arterial puncture can still occur. Performing the procedure in a dynamic fashion in the long-axis approach can help reduce the chances of accidental arterial puncture.[1,16]

Anatomy

IJ vein

The patient should be placed in a supine position, in slight Trendelenburg, to maximize venous return to the IJ with the head turned gently toward the contralateral shoulder. With too much head rotation, the sternocleidomastoid muscle can compress the underlying IJ and carotid artery.

Place the transducer parallel and superior to the clavicle, over the groove between the sternal and clavicular heads of the sternocleidomastoid muscle (**Fig. 7**). This procedure is one of the few instances in which the probe is placed so that the indicator is pointing toward the patient's left shoulder and not toward the right. The orientation marker on the screen is still to the upper left of the image. Visualize the IJ vein and carotid artery just deep to the sternocleidomastoid muscle. The IJ vein can be cannulated below the bifurcation of the sternal and clavicular heads of the sternocleidomastoid. In most patients, the IJ vein courses laterally and superficial to the carotid artery

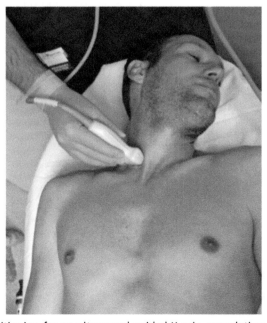

Fig. 7. Patient positioning for an ultrasound-guided IJ vein cannulation.

(**Fig. 8**). However, this relationship can change with head positioning and, in many patients, anatomic variability is present.[15] The IJ vein should compress easily under pressure from the probe and should increase in size with Valsalva maneuvers (**Fig. 9**).

Femoral vein

Place the patient in a supine position, in slight reverse Trendelenburg, with the leg and hip externally rotated. Place the transducer in a transverse plane just below the medial aspect of the inguinal ligament half way between the iliac wing and the pubic symphysis. The femoral vein can be seen medial to the femoral artery (**Fig. 10**). Use ultrasound to map out the course of both vessels before attempting the procedure. The femoral artery overlaps the femoral vein at some point in its anatomy in 65% of cases.[17] The puncture should occur below the inguinal ligament to prevent hemorrhage into the pelvis or accidental puncture of organs and intestines above the inguinal ligament.

Subclavian vein

Place the patient in supine position, in slight Trendelenburg, with the head rotated gently toward the contralateral side. Either the supraclavicular or infraclavicular approach can be used to access the subclavian vein. Cannulation of the subclavian vein can be performed in a static or dynamic fashion.

In the supraclavicular approach, place the transducer parallel to and above the medial clavicle (**Fig. 11**). Find the IJ vein and then fan and slide the probe inferiorly until the IJ joins the subclavian vein. At their juncture, there should be a large venous pool (**Fig. 12**). An oblique probe orientation may be required to obtain the best imaging of this confluence.

It is also possible to visualize the subclavian vein via the infraclavicular approach. The probe is positioned in a longitudinal fashion just below the clavicle with the beams angled in the cranial direction. The dark, anechoic subclavian vein is seen superior to the subclavian artery in this transverse, long-axis plane.

Technique

- Use a high-frequency linear array transducer to assess the potential sites for central venous access before choosing a vein for cannulation.

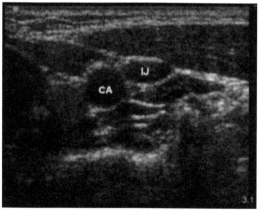

Fig. 8. Left IJ vein coursing lateral and superficial to the carotid artery (CA).

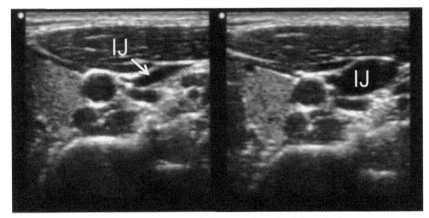

Fig. 9. Increase in IJ size from baseline (left image) and with Valsalva maneuvers (right image).

- Assess for any intraluminal clot or large proximal valves that may impair cannulation attempts.
- If an intraluminal clot is suspected (the vessel fails the compression test or a hyperechoic clot is visualized in the vessel lumen), attempt to obtain central venous access at another site.
- Place the patient in a position of comfort that maximizes venous return to the target vein and maneuvers the target vein into an easily accessible position (**Fig. 13**).
- Don sterile gear and prep and drape the patient and the ultrasound probe in a sterile fashion. Gel in direct contact with the ultrasound transducer does not need to be sterile. Reserve the sterile gel for use between the sterile probe cover and the patient's skin.
- Use the sterile ultrasound transducer to map out and identify the optimal cannulation site on the target vein.
- Inject local anesthetic using ultrasound guidance to ensure that the anesthetic is not accidentally injected into the vessel lumen.
- Center the target vein on the middle of the screen and obtain a long-axis view of the target vessel.

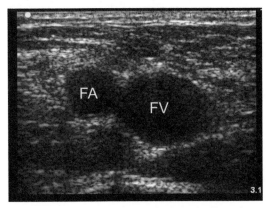

Fig. 10. Femoral vein (FV) lying medial to femoral artery (FA) on ultrasound.

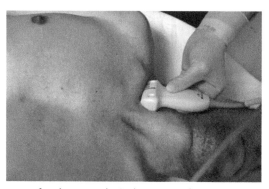

Fig. 11. Probe placement for the supraclavicular approach to accessing the subclavian vein.

- Under direct ultrasound guidance, puncture the skin with the needle. Watch the needle tip enter the vein through the proximal vessel wall (see **Fig. 4**). Aspirate back venous blood gently to ensure that the vein is patent.
- Continue placement of a central venous catheter using the Seldinger technique.
- Watch the guidewire insertion into the vein on a long-axis view. The guidewire can inadvertently puncture the posterior wall of the vein and cause accidental cannulation of adjacent vessels or tissue.
- Once the catheter has been secured, use ultrasound to assess for saline flushes through all available ports. Injection of saline can be seen as a swirling of bubbles within an enlarging vessel lumen.

Tips

- If you meet resistance during insertion of the guidewire, dilator, or catheter, do not continue to forcibly advance the wire or catheter because you may cause inadvertent vessel dissection. Use ultrasound to determine why resistance is being encountered (eg, vessel narrowing or stenosis, vessel thrombosis, insertion against the back wall of the vessel).

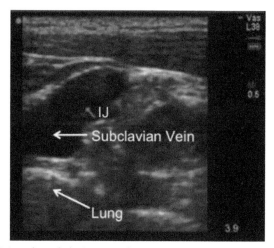

Fig. 12. IJ vein joining the subclavian vein from a supraclavicular approach.

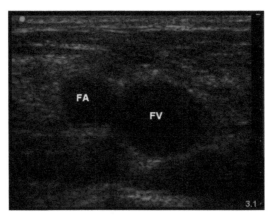

Fig. 13. External rotation of the hip and leg helps to separate the FA from the FV before cannulation attempts.

- Use the thumb of a large sterile glove if no commercial sterile probe cover is available.
- A clot may be present if a vein fails the compressibility test. In the acute phase, blood clots may be isoechoic to the surrounding blood and may not be visible on ultrasound. If the vein does not compress, attempt central venous access at a different site.

ULTRASOUND-GUIDED ARTERIAL ACCESS
Clinical Indications

Arterial access is indicated for continuous hemodynamic monitoring, frequent arterial blood gas (ABG) sampling, and failure of noninvasive monitoring methods.[3] Ultrasound should be used in difficult patients such as patients with systolic blood pressure less than 90 mm Hg, vasopressor use, pitting edema at the insertion site, previous attempts of ABGs at the site, or those with faint or nonpalpable pulses.[18] Ultrasound guidance for arterial access has higher success rates, reduced number of attempts, reduced number of catheters used, and decreased time to cannulation.[19–22]

Arterial lines may be placed in the radial, brachial, femoral, or dorsalis pedis arteries. The ulnar artery is less desirable because of its smaller size and close proximity to the ulnar nerve. The most common complications from arterial line placement are loss of blood flow caused by thrombosis and bleeding. Radial and femoral arteries are the preferred sites because of good collateral blood flow and easy compressibility.[3]

Anatomy: Radial Artery

Place the patient's upper extremity in anatomic position without rotation. Immobilize the wrist in dorsiflexion at 60° with padding underneath the wrist. Place a high-frequency linear array transducer over the distal wrist and slide it toward the radial aspect of the forearm until you can see the radial artery in the center of the ultrasound screen (**Fig. 14**). The radial artery is visualized as an echo-free, thick-walled, pulsatile structure located on the radial side of the wrist superficial to the flexor digitorum superficialis, flexor pollicis longus, and pronator quadratus.[11] Anatomic variation exists in the radial artery in 30% of cases.[23] Instead of performing the Allen test to check

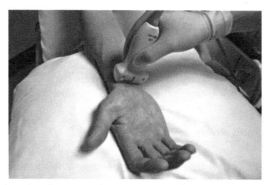

Fig. 14. Ultrasound probe placement for assessment of the radial artery. Begin midline on the wrist and slide the probe toward the radial aspect of the distal wrist until the radial artery is visualized.

for collateral flow, ultrasound can be used to assess for patency of the ulnar artery in the distal wrist.

Anatomy: Femoral Artery

The femoral artery can be palpated midway between the pubic symphysis and the anterior iliac spine. It should be cannulated distal to the inguinal ligament where it is compressible against the femoral head. It bifurcates into the superficial femoral artery and deep femoral artery distal to the inguinal ligament. In most patients, the femoral artery courses in between the lateral femoral nerve and medial femoral vein (**Fig. 15**). The femoral artery overlaps the femoral vein at some point in its anatomy in 65% of cases.[17]

To evaluate the femoral artery, place the ultrasound transducer in a transverse fashion just below the inguinal ligament. Identify the pulsatile, thick-walled, noncompressible femoral artery. If the patient is profoundly hypotensive, the femoral artery may be compressible on ultrasound. If chest compressions are being performed and no pulse is present, the femoral vein may pulsate with compressions. It is important to distinguish between the thinner-walled, oval-shaped femoral vein and the thicker-walled, round femoral artery.[3]

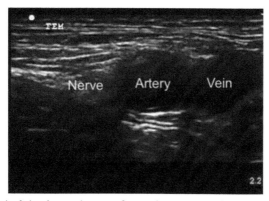

Fig. 15. Ultrasound of the femoral nerve, femoral artery, and femoral vein.

Anatomy: Brachial Artery

The brachial artery can be cannulated for arterial monitoring, but it is not an optimal site because there is no collateral circulation. The brachial artery is a continuation of the axially artery and bifurcates into the radial and ulnar arteries at the level of the radial head. When accessing the brachial artery, it should be punctured just proximal to the antecubital fossa where it overlies the brachialis muscle, avoiding the median and ulnar nerves (**Fig. 16**).

Anatomy: Dorsalis Pedis Artery

The dorsalis pedis artery is a continuation of the anterior tibial artery and lies in the subcutaneous tissue of the dorsal midfoot between the extensor hallucis longus tendon and the extensor digitorum longus. It is normally absent in 10% of patients. Collateral flow may be compromised by vascular disease. It is also prone to dislodgement in ambulatory patients. If the dorsalis pedis artery is used for hemodynamic monitoring, it is important to remember that blood pressure readings may be higher in this artery.[3]

Technique

- Perform a bedside ultrasound assessment with a high-frequency transducer to determine the optimal artery for cannulation. Find a large and superficial artery without overlying scar tissue.
- Use color Doppler or pulsed wave Doppler to identify arterial versus venous flow.
- Place the patient in a position of comfort with the access site properly exposed.
- Assemble the monitoring equipment and arterial line kit.
- Don sterile gear and prep and drape the patient and ultrasound probe in a sterile fashion.
- Inject local anesthetic around the target artery under ultrasound guidance to prevent accidental injection into the vessel lumen.
- Center the target artery on the ultrasound screen.
- Insert the needle underneath the center of the ultrasound probe at a 30° to 45° angle above the skin surface. Monitor the needle trajectory with in-plane visualization on ultrasound as you advance the needle into the arterial lumen.
- Once a flash has been obtained, make sure the needle has not punctured the posterior wall of the artery.
- Advance the catheter over the needle and connect the catheter to the arterial line tubing. Confirm and assess the arterial wave form on the monitor.

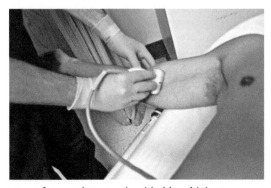

Fig. 16. Probe placement for an ultrasound-guided brachial artery cannulation.

Tips

- Apply local anesthesia sparingly because it may distort anatomy. Some experts recommend against injecting local anesthetic for this reason.
- In-plane, long-axis ultrasound guidance is optimal because it allows the user to visualize the needle tip puncturing the proximal wall of the artery.[18]
- Applying too much pressure with the ultrasound probe may impair blood flow distally during the procedure.
- A pediatric central venous access kit can be used for arterial monitoring in obese patients. The longer catheter is less likely to kink during insertion and manipulation.[18]

ULTRASOUND-GUIDED SUPRAPUBIC ASPIRATION
Clinical Indications

Suprapubic aspiration is the gold standard for sterile urine cultures in patients less than 2 years of age. This procedure decreases contamination by bypassing urethral contamination.[24] In adults, suprapubic aspiration can be used to decompress the bladder in cases of urinary retention, urethral trauma, urethral stricture, or known false passage. Complications of suprapubic aspiration include bowel perforation, accidental puncture of adjacent structures, hematuria, and unsuccessful aspiration. Bedside ultrasound should be used to determine whether the urinary bladder is adequately filled for aspiration, to identify anatomic abnormalities or variants, to reduce the risk of complications, and to guide needle aspiration.[11]

Anatomy

In the adult, the bladder is a pelvic organ. In the neonate, the bladder lies within the abdominal cavity. It is normally midline but is occasionally displaced laterally by abdominal or pelvic masses. On ultrasound, the normal bladder appears as an anechoic structure with a well-defined, hyperechoic muscular wall (**Fig. 17**).

Technique

- Visualize the bladder using a low-frequency or high-frequency transducer, depending on the patient's size and body habitus. In most adults, use the low-frequency curvilinear transducer. In most children, the high-frequency linear array transducer provides the best images during a bladder aspiration.

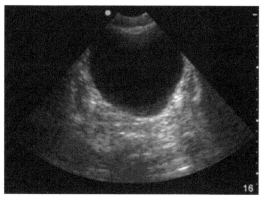

Fig. 17. Ultrasound of a normal bladder.

- Place the transducer in a transverse fashion just superior to the pubic symphysis (**Fig. 18**).
- The urinary bladder appears as an anechoic structure with posterior enhancement in both the longitudinal and transverse planes (see **Fig. 17**).
- Measure the bladder diameter in 3 planes: anteroposterior, transverse, and cranial-caudal. Multiple these three values by 0.52 to calculate the bladder volume.
- Use transverse diameter or total bladder volume to determine whether enough urine is present for aspiration. A transverse diameter of 1 to 3.5 cm or a total bladder volume of 10 mL is adequate for a successful bladder aspiration.[11,25]
- Repeat the scan every 15 minutes until enough fluid is present for aspiration.[25]
- Use ultrasound to determine the length of the needle required to successfully puncture the anterior bladder wall. Depth markers are typically seen on the right side of the ultrasound image.
- Once there is enough urine noted in the bladder on ultrasound, prep and drape the patient and the ultrasound probe in a sterile fashion.
- Inject local anesthetic under direct ultrasound guidance.
- Insert the needle under direct ultrasound visualization approximately 1 cm cranial to the pubic symphysis (**Fig. 19**).[24]
- If an indwelling suprapubic catheter is being placed, use ultrasound to guide and confirm catheter positioning in the urinary bladder (**Fig. 20**).

Tips

- Large ovarian cysts and distended bowel loops can be mistaken for the urinary bladder on ultrasound. Obtain multiple views of the structure and try to visualize urethral jets to confirm that you are looking at the bladder (**Fig. 21**). Peristalsis may be observed in bowel loops. Color flow is seen on Doppler imaging of the ovarian tissue surrounding a large ovarian cyst.[11]
- Avoid applying too much pressure with the probe in neonates, because this irritates the bladder and causes the neonate to urinate before the aspiration attempt.

ULTRASOUND-GUIDED ABSCESS LOCALIZATION FOR INCISION AND DRAINAGE
Clinical Indications

Ultrasound can be used to characterize soft tissue infections whenever there is suspicion of abscess formation. Ultrasound is more sensitive and specific than physical examination for detecting soft tissue abscesses.[26,27]

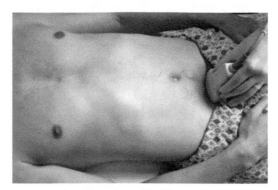

Fig. 18. Probe placement to view the urinary bladder.

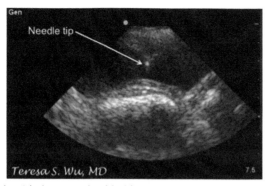

Fig. 19. Ultrasound-guided suprapubic bladder aspiration.

If the patient has a soft tissue cellulitis, ultrasound of that area shows a cobblestone appearance of the inflammatory fluid coursing between the soft tissue (**Fig. 22**). Because fluid accumulates within the cellulitic tissue, a phlegmon, or early abscess, may be seen on ultrasound (**Fig. 23**). Placing pressure with the probe over a phlegmon may cause the fluid contents to dissipate into the surrounding tissue. Once an abscess has formed, it appears as a hypoechoic fluid collection, with or without internal loculations or debris, surrounded by a brightly hyperechoic wall (**Fig. 24**). Applying color Doppler over the pocket of fluid should not show any color flow within the lumen of the abscess. Remember that other fluid collections such as a Baker cyst, hematoma, or vascular structures, can appear similar to abscesses on ultrasound. Color Doppler or pulsed wave Doppler imaging may be required to make the distinction.[9]

Technique

- Choose the appropriate ultrasound probe based on the location of the suspected fluid collection. High-frequency probes provide the best resolution, at the expense of penetration. Lower frequency probes should be used to visualize deeper structures.
- Place a Tegaderm over the probe face to minimize transmission of infections.

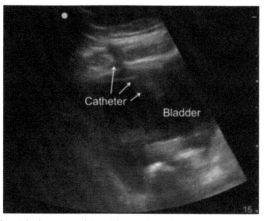

Fig. 20. Ultrasound-guided suprapubic catheter insertion.

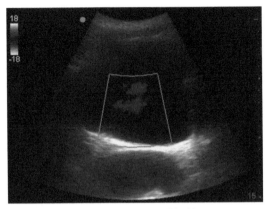

Fig. 21. Urethral jets visualized in a normal urinary bladder.

- Place the probe over the area of concern. Evaluate for the presence of cellulitis, phlegmon formation, or abscess. Obtain multiple views of the target structure to determine the depth and dimensions of the abscess pocket and visualize any loculations present.
- Carefully identify important surrounding structures such as blood vessels, nerves, muscles, tendons, and bone.
- Mark the site of the anticipated incision.
- Proceed with the incision and drainage.
- Use ultrasound after the procedure to ensure that all internal contents have been expressed.

Tips

- Use a water bath as an acoustic window if the area to be scanned is painful to touch. Float the ultrasound probe gently over the water bath to visualize the structures lying within the water.
- Apply color Doppler over all hypoechoic structures to ensure that the target structure is not a vessel or pseudoaneurysm.
- Note surrounding organs and neurovascular structures with ultrasound to prevent accidental incision or puncture during the procedure.

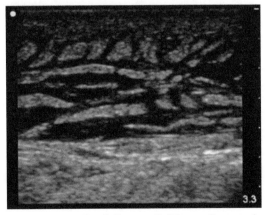

Fig. 22. Cobblestone appearance of soft tissue cellulitis on ultrasound.

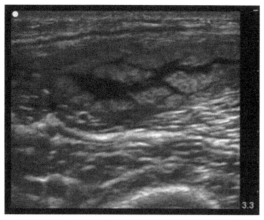

Fig. 23. Phlegmon or early abscess as depicted on bedside ultrasound. Note that the fluid collection is not clearly defined.

ULTRASOUND-GUIDED FOREIGN BODY LOCALIZATION
Clinical Indications

Retained foreign bodies can result in infection and morbidity if not removed in the acute phase.[28] Plain radiographs only reliably identify radiopaque glass and metal. Ultrasound can be used to visualize radiolucent foreign bodies such as wood, plastic, fish bones, and cactus spines with high sensitivity.[29–31] Ultrasound can be used to localize the foreign body and identify surrounding vascular structures to assist with operative planning and easy removal of the foreign material.

Most foreign bodies appear as hyperechoic structures on ultrasound. Acoustic shadowing may be present behind stone, wood, or plastic to variable degrees (**Fig. 25**). Reverberation artifact or comet tails may be seen with glass or metal foreign bodies (**Fig. 26**). In addition, there may be inflammatory hypoechoic fluid collections surrounding the foreign body (**Fig. 27**), which is called the halo sign and may represent edema, abscess, or granulation tissue. It is more common when presentation is delayed greater than 24 hours. Air may be visualized in the tract of the foreign body

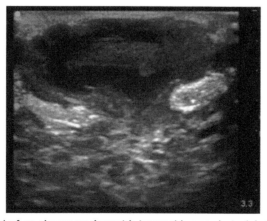

Fig. 24. Ultrasound of an abscess pocket with internal hyperechoic debris.

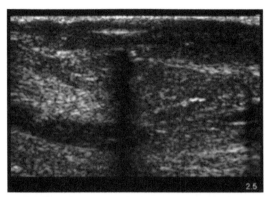

Fig. 25. Plastic foreign body with acoustic shadowing seen on ultrasound.

or hematomas may be visualized with or without clot as anechoic areas surrounding the foreign body. Wood eventually decomposes and loses echogenicity over time.[9,31]

Ultrasound evaluation is subject to false-positives and false-negatives. Limitations to ultrasound-guided foreign body removal include the anatomic site of puncture, type of foreign body being evaluated, instrumentation, overlying air bubbles, ultrasound beam width, size of the foreign body, and mobility of the foreign body.[32] If a comprehensive scan of the area is not performed, a second foreign body can easily be missed.[30]

Technique

- Choose an ultrasound transducer based on the location of the potential foreign body. High-frequency probes provide the best resolution, at the expense of penetration. Lower frequency probes should be used to visualize deeper structures.
- Use a lot of acoustic gel or place the patient's affected extremity in a water bath to create the best acoustic window. Radiographs may help guide where to begin the scan (**Fig. 28**).

Tips

- Have the patient identify the exact spot where the foreign body may have punctured the skin, and begin the scan there.

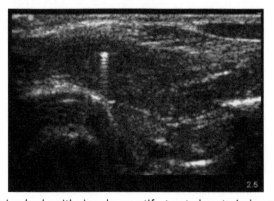

Fig. 26. Metal foreign body with ring-down artifact noted posteriorly on ultrasound.

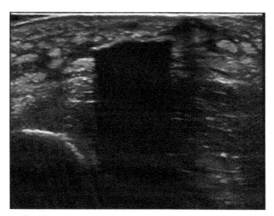

Fig. 27. Wood foreign body with prominent posterior acoustic shadowing. Note the edema and inflammatory changes in the surrounding tissue.

- Scan through the area methodically in multiple planes.
- Use a lot of gel or immerse the extremity in a water bath to enhance visualization of the foreign body.
- Assess for artifacts that may result from the presence of a foreign body (eg, ring-down artifact, posterior shadowing, surrounding edema)

ULTRASOUND-GUIDED ARTHROCENTESIS
Clinical Indications

Synovial fluid analysis is required to differentiate a septic joint form other painful inflammatory monoarthropathies. Synovial fluid analysis with a positive culture, white blood cell count greater than 250,000/mL and greater than 90% polymorphonuclear cells are the only reliable laboratory findings associated with a septic joint.[33] If a septic joint is suspected, early drainage and initiation of antibiotics can prevent further joint destruction and minimize the need for more invasive procedures.[34] Relieving pressure on the joint capsule caused by the effusion results in immediate pain relief and should be considered in all patients presenting with a joint effusion and pain.[35,36]

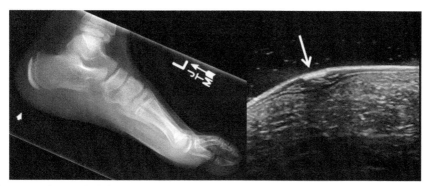

Fig. 28. Radiograph (*left*) and ultrasound image (*right*) of an embedded wooden toothpick in a patient's heel. Note that the radiograph does not show the foreign body. Water bath ultrasound was used to help identify the foreign body location. Both the *arrowhead* (*left*) and the *arrow* (*right*) identify the location of the foreign body. (*Courtesy of* M. Connell, MD, Phoenix, AZ.)

An ultrasound-guided arthrocentesis decreases time required for the procedure, minimizes patient pain, increases success rate, and decreases complications.[7,37] Ultrasound guidance can be used during arthrocentesis of any major joint. The following sections explains how to perform an ultrasound-guided arthrocentesis of some of the major joints.

Anatomy

Knee

Position the patient supine with knee slightly flexed over a supporting towel or roll of sheets. Use a high-frequency linear array transducer. Scan along the medial and lateral aspects of the knee to determine where the largest pocket of fluid is visualized (**Figs. 29** and **30**).

A knee effusion is most easily visible in the lateral and medial recesses of the suprapatellar bursa, which is an extension of the knee joint. It is surrounded superiorly by the quadriceps muscle, and inferiorly by the femur. The normal joint has less than 2 mm of fluid visible on ultrasound (**Fig. 31**).[3] An effusion may be hypoechoic or hyperechoic, depending on the amount of inflammatory debris present, and may contain loculations or septations. Traumatic effusions may contain clotted blood and appear more hyperechoic than inflammatory effusions (**Fig. 32**). Do not confuse a joint effusion with prepatellar bursitis, in which fluid is seen anterior to the patella, or a Baker cyst, in which fluid is visualized as a beaklike collection in the posterior fossa of the knee.[11]

Hip

Place the patient in a supine position with the knee in slight flexion and the hip in slight internal rotation. This position displaces the joint fluid anteriorly.[35] A high-frequency probe should be used in thin patients, whereas a lower frequency probe may be required in large or obese patients. Scan the contralateral, normal hip first to obtain baseline images. Place the transducer along the long axis of the hip inferior to the inguinal ligament and lateral to the femoral vessels. A sagittal oblique orientation of the probe provides the best views of the hip. Visualize the hyperechoic convex femoral head, and hyperechoic concave femoral neck. The articular cartilage is a thin hypoechoic line adjacent to the cortex of the femoral head, and the acetabular labrum is medial and superior to the femoral head (**Fig. 33**).

The joint capsule extends from the acetabular labrum to its insertion at the base of the femoral neck. An effusion typically appears as a hypoechoic fluid collection

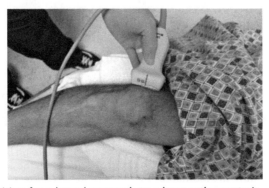

Fig. 29. Probe position for a lateral approach to a knee arthrocentesis.

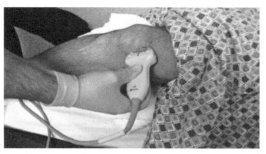

Fig. 30. Probe position for a medial approach to a knee arthrocentesis.

elevating the joint capsule most prominently in the anterior synovial recess, anterior to the femoral neck (**Fig. 34**). A pathologic effusion is present when you see a fluid stripe greater than 5 mm, or greater than 2 mm compared with the asymptomatic, contralateral hip, at the widest anteroposterior dimension between the femoral neck and joint capsule.[38]

To perform an ultrasound-guided hip aspiration, orient the transducer in a transverse fashion and identify the femoral nerve, artery, and vein just medial to the hip joint. Enter the skin 2.5 cm (1 inch) lateral to the femoral artery, 2.5 cm below the inguinal ligament. Obtain a long-axis view of the needle entering the joint fluid from a lateral approach.

Ankle
Position the patient's ankle in slight plantar flexion or allow the ankle to hang freely over the side of the bed or chair. Using a high-frequency linear array transducer, scan in the sagittal plane over the distal tibia (**Fig. 35**). Move the transducer distally until the anterior synovial recess of the joint appears as a V shape formed by the distal tibia superiorly and the talar dome inferiorly. An intracapsular fat pad is typically seen here (**Fig. 36**). An effusion appears as a triangular, hypoechoic fluid collection greater than 3 mm in diameter, filling the V-shaped area. It appears more rectangular along the medial aspect of the joint. The joint capsule appears as an echogenic line bordering the effusion.

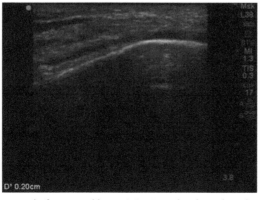

Fig. 31. Lateral ultrasound of a normal knee. It is normal to have less than 2 mm of anechoic fluid in the suprapatellar bursa.

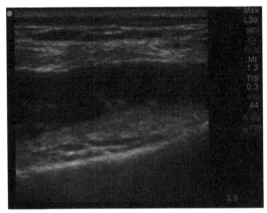

Fig. 32. An ultrasound image of a traumatic knee effusion. Note the hyperechoic clotted blood floating within the hypoechoic effusion.

The anterior tibial/dorsalis pedis artery courses along the medial joint. Identify it in a transverse view (**Fig. 37**) before attempting aspiration. Aspiration can be performed in a static or dynamic fashion. If aspiration is performed in a static fashion, avoid the dorsalis pedis artery by using a lateral approach.

Shoulder: anterior approach

Place the patient in a seated position, with the arm extended in slight abduction and the palm facing up. Place a high-frequency probe in a transverse fashion over the anterior shoulder at the level of the coracoid process (**Fig. 38**). Identify the deltoid muscle deep to the skin and soft tissue. Visualize the large, smooth, hyperechoic humeral head and the anterior surface of the medial, flatter, hyperechoic coracoid process (**Fig. 39**). Cartilage surrounding the humeral head appears hypoechoic. A joint effusion is seen accumulating between the humeral head and coracoid process anteriorly.

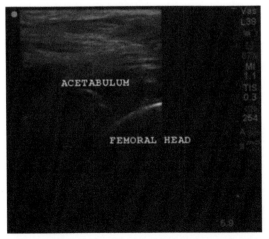

Fig. 33. An ultrasound of a normal hip. The acetabulum is nearfield to the femoral head. Note the normal hypoechoic articular cartilage overlying the femoral head.

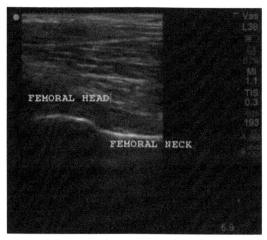

Fig. 34. Ultrasound of a normal hip. Note that the anterior recess overlies the femoral neck underneath the joint capsule where an effusion will accumulate.

For an anterior arthrocentesis of the shoulder, place the transducer in a transverse fashion and identify the V-shaped recess between the coracoid process and the humeral head. To perform the procedure in a dynamic fashion, insert the needle 1 to 2 cm inferior and lateral to the coracoid process and watch the needle tip enter the effusion.

Shoulder: posterior approach
Position the patient with the elbow flexed and the forearm at the patient's side in neutral position. Place a high-frequency linear array transducer in a transverse fashion, posterior to the shoulder, just below the acromion (**Fig. 40**). Visualize the posterior deltoid muscle deep to the skin and subcutaneous tissue. The triangular, hypoechoic infraspinatus muscle and hyperechoic tendon is deep to the deltoid muscle and points laterally over the curved hyperechoic humeral head. Normal surrounding cartilage appears as a thin hyperechoic line around the bony cortex. Locate the hyperechoic glenoid rim superficial and medial to the humeral head, and the hyperechoic scapula medial and deep to the humeral head (**Fig. 41**). An effusion appears as an anechoic

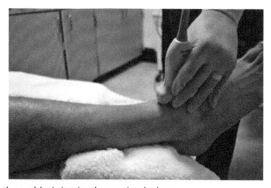

Fig. 35. Scanning the ankle joint in the sagittal plane.

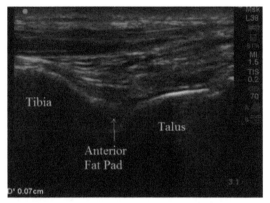

Fig. 36. Ultrasound of a normal ankle joint. A fat pad is noted in the ankle joint surrounded by the tibia and talar dome.

collection of fluid in the groove between the humeral head and the dorsal glenoid rim. Subacromial bursitis produces hypoechoic fluid beneath the deltoid muscle, but superior to the supraspinatus tendon. It can be confused with an effusion but is not present in an anterior view of the shoulder.

To perform a posterior arthrocentesis of the shoulder, place the transducer transversely across the posterior shoulder and tilt the lateral edge of the transducer slightly inferiorly to obtain an optimal view of the joint. Locate the effusion filling the groove between the humeral head and glenoid labrum. Obtain a long-axis view of the needle entering the joint space via a lateral approach. The needle should be seen entering the joint capsule along the medial border of the humeral head to avoid the circumflex scapular vessels and suprascapular nerve coursing just medial to the glenoid rim.[11]

Elbow
The patient should be seated with the elbow flexed at 90° and forearm in neutral position. Use a high-frequency linear array transducer and scan in a longitudinal or oblique fashion around the triangle formed by the lateral epicondyle, radial head, and olecranon process (**Fig. 42**). The humerus appears as an echogenic flat line that forms a U-shaped depression distally corresponding with the olecranon fossa (**Fig. 43**). This space normally contains the hyperechoic posterior fat pad. An effusion appears as a

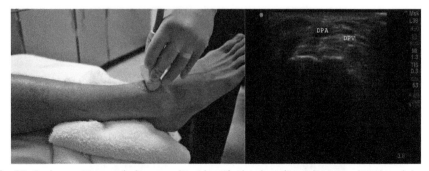

Fig. 37. Probe position and ultrasound to identify the dorsalis pedis artery (DPA) and dorsalis pedis vein (DPV).

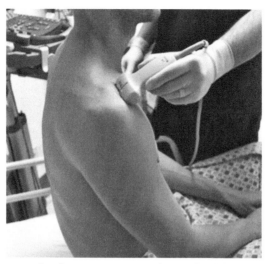

Fig. 38. Probe placement for the anterior approach to a shoulder aspiration.

hypoechoic or anechoic fluid collection pushing the fat pad superiorly and distending the joint capsule posteriorly.

Elbow aspiration can be performed in a static or dynamic fashion. Scan around until the largest fluid collection is identified. A lateral approach avoids adjacent nerves and tendons that surround the joint effusion during the procedure.

Technique for an Ultrasound-guided Arthrocentesis

- Place the patient in a position of comfort with the target joint exposed.
- Scan around the joint and identify the area that provides the best, direct access to the largest collection of joint fluid.
- Identify surrounding vessels, nerves, tendons, and muscles.
- Don sterile gear and prep and drape the patient and the ultrasound probe in a sterile fashion.

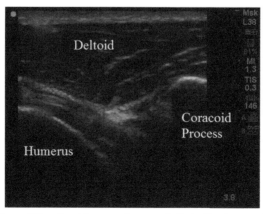

Fig. 39. Anterior view of the shoulder on ultrasound. Note the hyperechoic humeral head and coracoid process.

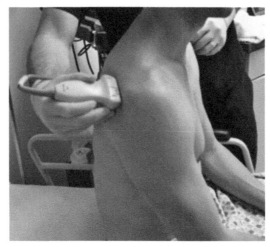

Fig. 40. Probe position for a posterior shoulder arthrocentesis.

- Administer local anesthetic under direct ultrasound guidance.
- Insert the needle and monitor its trajectory into the joint effusion using a long-axis approach (**Fig. 44**).
- Aspirate the desired amount of fluid for symptomatic relief and diagnostic purposes.

Tips

- Use ultrasound to manipulate the joint space into the position that provides the best access to the effusion.
- Always scan the contralateral, asymptomatic joint for a comparison of the sonographic structures.
- Squeeze the joint manually during aspiration to move the effusion toward the needle and increase the amount of fluid removed.
- Administering local anesthetic under ultrasound guidance into the joint space after arthrocentesis can control pain for several hours.

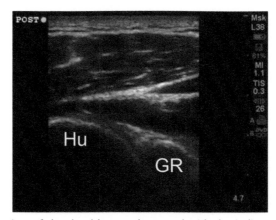

Fig. 41. Posterior view of the shoulder on ultrasound with the indicator marker oriented laterally. Note the hyperechoic humeral head (Hu) and hyperechoic glenoid rim (GR).

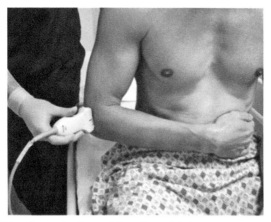

Fig. 42. Probe position for evaluation of the elbow joint.

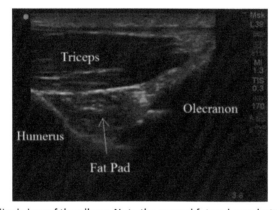

Fig. 43. Longitudinal view of the elbow. Note the normal fat pad seen between the humerus and olecranon.

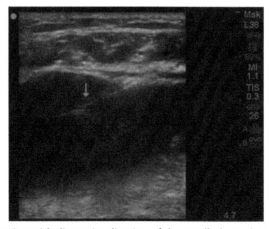

Fig. 44. Joint aspiration with direct visualization of the needle (*arrow*) entering the joint on bedside ultrasound.

SUMMARY

Ultrasound guidance can be used in a wide variety of bedside procedures. It enables real-time visualization of the surrounding anatomy while performing the procedure, therefore increasing safety, saving time, and minimizing complications. As experience and comfort with ultrasound grow, so too will its use in the completion of standard bedside procedures.

REFERENCES

1. Lamperti M, Bodenham AR, Pittiruti M, et al. International evidence-based recommendations on ultrasound-guided vascular access. Intensive Care Med 2012; 38(7):1105–17.
2. Riley DC, Garcia S. Emergency department ultrasonography guided long-axis antecubital intravenous cannulation: how to do it. Crit Ultrasound J 2012;4(1):3.
3. Roberts JR, Hedges JR. Clinical procedures in emergency medicine. 5th edition. Philadelphia: Elsevier; 2010. ISBN 978–1416036234.
4. Gillette JF, Susini J. Deep brachial vein catheterization for total parenteral nutrition–an alternate approach: review of 154 cases. JPEN J Parenter Enteral Nutr 1984;8(1):49–50.
5. Bauman M, Braude D, Crandall C. Ultrasound-guidance vs. standard technique in difficult vascular access patients by ED technicians. Am J Emerg Med 2009; 27(2):135–40.
6. Costantino TG, Parikh AK, Satz WA, et al. Ultrasonography-guided peripheral intravenous access versus traditional approaches in patients with difficult intravenous access. Ann Emerg Med 2005;46(5):456–61.
7. Wu TS, Stefanski P. Basic ultrasound-guided procedures. Emergency medicine reports. The Practical Journal for Emergency Physicians 2011;32(5):1–16.
8. Dargin JM, Rebholz CM, Lowenstein RA, et al. Ultrasonography-guided peripheral intravenous catheter survival in ED patients with difficult access. Am J Emerg Med 2010;28(1):1–7.
9. Simon RR, Hoffman JR, Smith M. Modified new approaches for rapid intravenous access. Ann Emerg Med 1987;16(1):44–9.
10. Witting MD, Schenkel SM, Lawner BJ, et al. Effects of vein width and depth on ultrasound-guided peripheral intravenous success rates. J Emerg Med 2010; 39(1):70–5.
11. Ma JO, Mateer JR, Blaivas M. Emergency ultrasound. 2nd edition. New York: McGraw-Hill; 2008. ISBN 978-0-07-147904-2.
12. Rothschild JM. Making health care safer: a critical analysis of patient safety practices. No 43. Rockville (MD): Agency for Healthcare Research and Quality; 2001. p. 245–53 AHRQ publication no 01-E058. Ultrasound guidance of central vein catheterization: evidence report/technology assessment.
13. ACS Committee on Perioperative Care. Revised statement on recommendations for use of real-time ultrasound guidance for placement of central venous catheters. Bull Am Coll Surg 2011;96(2):36–7.
14. Randolph AG, Cook DJ, Gonzales CA, et al. Ultrasound guidance for placement of central venous catheters: a meta-analysis of the literature. Crit Care Med 1996; 24(12):2053–8.
15. Karakitsos D, Labropoulos N, De Groot E, et al. Real-time ultrasound-guided catheterization of the internal jugular vein: a prospective comparison with the landmark technique in critical care patients. Crit Care 2006;10(6):R162.

16. Stone MB, Moon C, Sutijono D, et al. Needle tip visualization during ultrasound-guided vascular access: short-axis vs. long-axis approach. Am J Emerg Med 2010;28:343–7.
17. Baum PA, Matsumoto AH, Teitelbaum GP, et al. Anatomic relationship between the common femoral artery and vein: CT evaluation and clinical significance. Radiology 1989;173(3):775–7.
18. Hofmann LJ, Reha JL, Hetz SP. Ultrasound-guided arterial line catheterization in the critically ill: technique and review. J Vasc Access 2010;11(2):106–11.
19. Shiloh AL, Savel RH, Paulin LM, et al. Ultrasound-guided catheterization of the radial artery: a systematic review and meta-analysis of randomized controlled trials. Chest 2011;139(3):524–9.
20. Shiver S, Blaivas M, Lyon M. A prospective comparison of ultrasound-guided and blindly placed radial arterial catheters. Acad Emerg Med 2006;13(12):1275–9.
21. Tada T, Amagasa S, Horikawa H. Absence of efficacy of ultrasonic two-way Doppler flow detector in routine percutaneous arterial cannulation. J Anesth 2003;17(3):206–7.
22. Tada T, Amagasa S, Horikawa H. Usefulness of ultrasonic two-way Doppler flow detector in percutaneous arterial puncture in patients with hemorrhagic shock. J Anesth 2003;17(1):70–1.
23. McCormack LJ, Cauldwell EW, Anson BJ. Brachial and antebrachial arterial patterns; a study of 750 extremities. Surg Gynecol Obstet 1953;96(1):43–54.
24. Nagia S. Ultrasound guided suprapubic aspiration. Indian Pediatr 1998;35(8):807–9.
25. García-Nieto V, Navarro JF, Sánchez-Almeida E, et al. Standards for ultrasound guidance of suprapubic bladder aspiration. Pediatr Nephrol 1997;11(5):607–9.
26. Iverson K, Haritos D, Thomas R, et al. The effect of bedside ultrasound on diagnosis and management of soft tissue infections in a pediatric ED. Am J Emerg Med 2012;30(8):1347–51.
27. Sivitz AB, Lam SH, Ramirez-Schrempp D, et al. Effect of bedside ultrasound on management of pediatric soft-tissue infection. J Emerg Med 2010;39(5):637–43.
28. Halaas GW. Management of foreign bodies in the skin. Am Fam Physician 2007;76(5):683–8.
29. Saboo SS, Saboo SH, Soni SS, et al. High-resolution sonography is effective in detection of soft tissue foreign bodies: experience from a rural Indian center. J Ultrasound Med 2009;28(9):1245–9.
30. Nienaber A, Harvey M, Cave G. Accuracy of bedside ultrasound for the detection of soft tissue foreign bodies by emergency doctors. Emerg Med Australas 2010;22(1):30–4.
31. Mohammadi A, Ghasemi-Rad M, Khodabakhsh M. Non-opaque soft tissue foreign body: sonographic findings. BMC Med Imaging 2011;11:9.
32. Bradley M. Image-guided soft-tissue foreign body extraction - success and pitfalls. Clin Radiol 2012;67(6):531–4.
33. Margaretten ME, Kohlwes J, Moore D, et al. Does this adult patient have septic arthritis? JAMA 2007;297(13):1478–88.
34. Park AL, Dlabach JA. Infectious arthritis. Campbell's operative orthopaedics. St Louis (MO): Mosby; 2003. p. 687–700.
35. Berman L, Fink AM, Wilson D, et al. Technical note: identifying and aspirating hip effusions. Br J Radiol 1995;68(807):306–10.

36. Givon U, Liberman B, Schindler A, et al. Treatment of septic arthritis of the hip joint by repeated ultrasound-guided aspirations. J Pediatr Orthop 2004;24(3): 266–70.

37. Wiler JL, Costantino TG, Filippone L, et al. Comparison of ultrasound-guided and standard landmark techniques for knee arthrocentesis. J Emerg Med 2010;39(1): 76–82.

38. Freeman K, Dewitz A, Baker WE. Ultrasound-guided hip arthrocentesis in the ED. Am J Emerg Med 2007;25(1):80–6.

Advanced Ultrasound Procedures

Nicholas Hatch, MD[a],*, Teresa S. Wu, MD[b]

KEYWORDS

- Ultrasound guidance • Pericardiocentesis • Thoracentesis • Paracentesis
- Lumbar puncture • Nerve block • Peritonsillar abscess • Advanced procedures

KEY POINTS

- Ultrasound capabilities can assist in increasing the success and precision of many bedside procedures traditionally performed using landmark guidance alone.
- Ultrasound guidance is already becoming the standard of care in many bedside procedures, and providers should be familiar with its use in such applications.
- Procedures using ultrasound guidance described in this article include pericardiocentesis, thoracentesis, paracentesis, lumbar puncture, peripheral nerve blocks, and peritonsillar abscess drainage.
- Preparation is key. Knowledge of normal anatomy and associated abnormality, along with understanding of the procedure, necessary equipment, and associated complications can help lead to successful procedures while minimizing adverse outcomes.

ULTRASOUND-GUIDED PERICARDIOCENTESIS
Background

The heart is protected by 2 layers of pericardium called the visceral pericardium and the parietal pericardium. The visceral pericardium, which is immediately adherent to the epicardium, is surrounded by the parietal pericardium, a protective, fibrinous layer normally 2 mm thick. These 2 layers are normally well approximated and separated by less than 50 mL of pericardial fluid.

Any abnormal accumulation of fluid in this space creates a pericardial effusion. The clinical effects vary and are determined by the cause of the accumulation, the fluid type, and, most importantly, how quickly it develops.[1] Causes of pericardial effusion include hemorrhage, infection, malignant effusions, chronic pericarditis, autoimmune diseases, inflammatory processes, and other idiopathic causes.

Cardiac tamponade is a result of pressures within the pericardial space exceeding the right ventricular filling pressures, and represents a true cardiovascular emergency.

There are no disclosures to report.

[a] Department of Emergency Medicine, Maricopa Medical Center, 2601 East Roosevelt Street, Phoenix, AZ 85008, USA; [b] EM Residency Program, Department of Emergency Medicine, Maricopa Medical Center, University of Arizona College of Medicine-Phoenix, 2601 East Roosevelt Street, Phoenix, AZ 85008, USA
* Corresponding author.
E-mail address: hatchnr@gmail.com

Tamponade can develop with as little as 150 mL of fluid if it has accumulated rapidly. When the intrapericardial pressure exceeds the right ventricular pressure, ventricular filling is impaired, preload is reduced, and cardiac output decreases.

Traditionally, practitioners performing a pericardiocentesis relied on anatomic landmarks alone. This approach put the diaphragm, liver, gastrointestinal tract, lung, and myocardial tissue at risk for accidental perforation or laceration. Echocardiographic-guided pericardiocentesis using the subxiphoid approach is relatively safe and effective, with 97% success and only 1% having serious complications.[2] With ultrasound guidance, practitioners have improved complication rates and have discovered other approaches to performing a bedside pericardiocentesis.[1]

Diagnosis

Early stages of pericardial tamponade may produce signs and symptoms of dyspnea, positional relief with sitting forward, tachycardia, displaced point of maximal impulse, and narrowed pulse pressure. As tamponade becomes more severe, additional findings may include Beck's triad (muffled heart sounds, elevated jugular venous pressure, hypotension) and evidence of shock. Pulsus paradoxus may be a useful clue when it is present and detectable. Pain is usually not present until late tamponade occurs or if there is a concurrent pericarditis.

An electrocardiogram (ECG) is typically the first diagnostic test obtained, and may show findings such as low-voltage QRS complexes, PR-segment depression, and ST-segment elevation. Electrical alternans is commonly described, but is very insensitive and seen only in less than 20% of cases.

A chest radiograph may show an enlarged cardiac silhouette; however, this is usually not evident until effusions are moderately sized or larger. The pericardial fat pad sign may be seen on lateral views, and is described as a lucent interval between the anterior heart and the chest wall.

Bedside 2-dimensional cardiac ultrasonography is the best way of making the diagnosis of a pericardial effusion and cardiac tamponade in the critically ill patient, and can be used to guide an emergent bedside pericardiocentesis. Tamponade results as a pericardial effusion progressively increases in pressure. As the effusion develops, collapse of the right atrium during diastole will be the first sonographic change, and is highly sensitive for tamponade. Eventually pericardial pressures will overwhelm the right ventricle as well, and cause both the right atrium and right ventricle to collapse during diastole. This finding indicates more severe tamponade, and is more specific than right atrial collapse alone.[3] Once end-diastolic right ventricular collapse is noted on bedside ultrasonography, a pericardiocentesis must be performed immediately to release the pressure surrounding the heart.

Precautions

- Patients with a pericardial effusion with any indication of clinical deterioration and instability will need an emergent bedside pericardiocentesis performed before more definitive management.
- Pericardial effusions secondary to trauma or ventricular wall rupture will likely not stop bleeding spontaneously, and may have more complications with bedside drainage. In general, one should avoid performing a closed pericardiocentesis in these cases, and instead insert a catheter into the pericardial sac that allows for continuous or intermittent drainage of any blood or fluid that accumulates.
- In those presenting with hemodynamic instability, intravenous hydration may temporarily stabilize vital signs while preparing for the procedure. Half of patients

with tamponade show modest increases in cardiac output from a single 500-mL normal saline bolus.[4]

- Correct use of bedside echocardiography allows the provider to significantly reduce complications, and leads to a more rapid and safe technique for decompressing the pericardial effusion.
- Direct visualization of the cardiothoracic anatomy allows the provider to determine the best approach to perform the procedure (subxiphoid vs apical vs intercostal) while mapping out surrounding structures so as to minimize complications.[5]

Procedure

- Supplies needed for pericardiocentesis are listed in **Box 1**.
- Use a 5- to 1-MHz phased-array transducer or a 5- to 2-MHz curvilinear transducer. The phased-array transducer is the preferred probe because of its smaller footprint, which allows for easier manipulation in the subxiphoid region and intercostal spaces.
- Evaluate the effusion using subxiphoid, parasternal (intercostal), and apical views to determine the best approach for minimizing risk to adjacent structures (**Fig. 1**). Use the depth markers located on the side of the ultrasound screen to determine the depth from the skin to the pericardial space.
- Subxiphoid views are often the easiest to obtain and correlate with the traditional blind approach. Echocardiographic subxiphoid views are often superior to other approaches, owing to the acoustic window provided by liver tissue and the lack of overlying osseous structures (**Fig. 2**). Pericardiocentesis using this approach does carry an increased risk of liver puncture.[6]
- Parasternal (intercostal) views may allow direct access to the pericardium without any overlying organs being punctured. This approach does put important arterial structures at risk, however, including the internal mammary artery or the left anterior descending artery.[7]
- Apical views may be more difficult to obtain at the bedside, particularly in female or obese patients; however, they may give unobstructed access to the pericardium close to the chest wall. Adequate views are most commonly obtained

---

Box 1
Supplies needed for pericardiocentesis

Sterile drapes or towels

Sterile ultrasound transducer cover with sterile ultrasound gel

Chlorhexidine or appropriate skin antiseptic

Lidocaine 1% or 2% with epinephrine

Injection needle (25 gauge, 1.5 inch)

Pericardiocentesis needle or long 16- to 18-gauge needle (5–10 cm)

Three-way stopcock

5-mL and 20-mL or 60-mL Luer-lock syringes

Central venous access kit (if leaving catheter in pericardium)

No. 11 blade scalpel

Sterile gauze pads

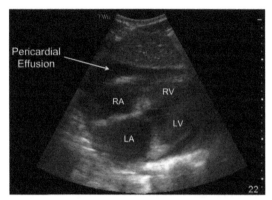

Fig. 1. Normal subxiphoid cardiac view. LA, left atrium; LV, left ventricle; RA, right atrium; RV, right ventricle. (*Courtesy of* T. Wu, MD, Phoenix, AZ.)

near the point of maximum impulse, located in the mid-axillary line at the sixth to seventh intercostal space (**Fig. 3**). This approach does carry an increased risk of iatrogenic pneumothorax.[8]

- Prepare and drape the patient in the usual fashion, including sterile preparation of the ultrasound transducer. Insert and advance the needle while maintaining gentle negative pressure with the syringe, taking care to monitor the trajectory and depth of the needle at all times.
- Continue advancement of the syringe with negative pressure until the needle tip is seen to enter the pericardial space and fluid or blood is aspirated (**Fig. 4**).
- Attach a 20- to 60-mL syringe to the stopcock and continue to aspirate fluid (50–200 mL) until there is resolution of the cardiac tamponade, as determined by vital signs or dynamic echocardiography.
- A catheter may be placed in the pericardial sac to allow for continuous drainage, using either a pericardiocentesis kit or a standard central venous catheter. Extended catheter drainage over several days may help to minimize recurrences.[9]
- Right ventricular volumes will typically improve by 77% after the removal of the first 200 mL of a pericardial effusion causing tamponade.[9]

Pearls and Pitfalls

- Although the phased-array transducer is preferred for this procedure in most patients, higher-frequency linear transducers (10–5 MHz) may provide better needle

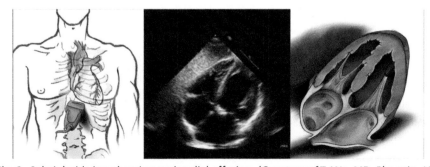

Fig. 2. Subxiphoid view showing pericardial effusion. (*Courtesy of* T. Wu, MD, Phoenix, AZ.)

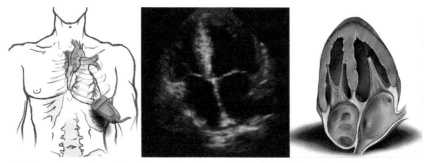

Fig. 3. Normal apical cardiac views. (*Courtesy of* T. Wu, MD, Phoenix, AZ.)

visualization. The phased-array or curvilinear transducer should be used initially to locate the largest fluid collection with the least obstructed point of access, at which point a linear probe can be used to complete the procedure guidance. Remember that higher-frequency probes, such as the linear-array transducer, sacrifice the ability to visualize deeper structures for the sake of improved resolution of shallow structures.

- The parasternal long-axis view offers the advantage of being able to monitor the entire trajectory of the needle throughout the paracentesis. Needle location can be confirmed in the pericardial space by injection of 1 to 2 mL of normal saline with direct ultrasonographic visualization of bubbling within the pericardial sac.
- Rapid pericardial decompression can cause a sudden increase in left ventricular preload, which may lead to adverse hemodynamic consequences such as flash pulmonary edema, circulatory collapse, bradycardia, or rebound hypertension.

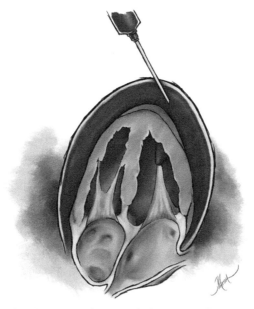

Fig. 4. Pericardiocentesis using an apical approach. (*Courtesy of* N. Hatch, MD, Phoenix, AZ.)

Remove just enough fluid to restore an adequate perfusing blood pressure while being mindful of potential complications.[9]
- Use ultrasound guidance to locate and visualize surrounding vascular structures. Avoid inadvertent puncture of the internal mammary artery, which lies 3 to 5 cm lateral to the sternal border, and the intercostal arteries that run along the lower rib margin.
- Evaluation of pericardial aspirate can assist with confirmation of correct placement. Intracardiac blood or traumatic effusions will clot, whereas blood that has transmigrated into the pericardial space will not because it is defibrinated. If unclear, inject a small amount of normal saline and visualize the distribution of the saline bubbles in the pericardial space.

ULTRASOUND-GUIDED THORACENTESIS
Background

The lungs are surrounded by pleura, a bilayered membrane that reflects on itself as it transitions from covering the outer surface of the lung (visceral pleura) to the inner surface of the chest wall (parietal pleura). A small amount of physiologic fluid is present to separate and lubricate the pleural surfaces. The lymphatic system normally drains circulating pleural fluid, at rates anywhere from 0.1 to 3.0 mL/kg/h.[10]

A pleural effusion develops with imbalance of Starling forces, changes in either membrane (pleural) permeability or driving pressures. Effusion becomes significant as the rate of accumulation exceeds rate of removal. As effusions increase in size, respiratory dynamics are compromised secondary to mass effect. Limited lung expansion can lead to atelectasis. Chronic effusions generally allow for compensation of respiratory dynamics, but provide their own complications such as secondary infections and local adhesions.

Diagnosis

Thoracentesis traditionally has relied on physical examination findings for localization of the effusion at the bedside. Physical examination traditionally utilizes auscultation, percussion, and tactile fremitus for the diagnosis, although sensitivity and specificity varies greatly depending on provider skill level and patient habitus. Egophony or a pleural friction rub may also be noted.

Chest radiographs are clearly most useful in initial presentation and diagnosis of a suspected effusion. Upright posteroanterior and lateral films will readily show effusions that are significant enough to impair respiratory dynamics. Lateral decubitus films may be useful if loculated effusions are suspected. Although other imaging modalities more commonly identify the presence and possible cause of the effusion, appearance on radiography or computed tomography (CT) cannot be used to reliably predict landmarks during a thoracentesis, as the effusion may redistribute with patient repositioning. Ultrasound guidance can both identify the presence of an effusion and define its location at the bedside (**Fig. 5**), allowing for increased success rates and fewer complications.[11]

Precautions

- Complications are primarily a result of direct injury to surrounding structures, such as the lung, spleen, liver, diaphragm, or ventricular wall of the heart. Ultrasound guidance has been shown to reduce these injuries when used appropriately at the bedside.[12]
- Consider transfusing blood products or factors before the procedure if a patient is thrombocytopenic or hypocoagulable (activated partial thromboplastin time

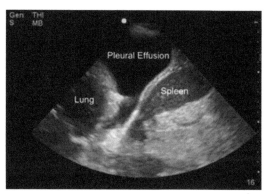

Fig. 5. Bedside ultrasonogram showing a significant left pleural effusion above the spleen. Note the excellent acoustic window provided by the effusion, and the echogenicity of the diaphragm. (*Courtesy of* T. Wu, MD, Phoenix, AZ.)

or prothrombin time greater than twice the normal limit, or a platelet count <50,000/mm^3).

- Rapid, large-volume thoracentesis should be avoided, as it can cause significant hypotension and reexpansion pulmonary edema. Limit initial fluid removal to 1000 to 1500 mL.[13] Patients with renal failure, uremia, or coagulation dysfunction are more likely to have acute reaccumulation of a pleural effusion following drainage, and should be monitored closely.
- Avoid puncturing through skin with any burns, cellulitis, or other infectious lesions.

Procedure

- Supplies needed for thoracentesis are listed in **Box 2**.
- Use a 5- to 1-MHz phased-array transducer or a 5- to 2-MHz curvilinear transducer to visualize the pleural effusion and surrounding structures. The phased-array transducer is preferred because of its smaller footprint, which allows for easier manipulation in the intercostal spaces.
- Ideally the patient should be upright, in a seated position, leaning forward, and resting on a bedside table. The insertion site is most commonly in the mid-scapular line or the posterior axillary line. Additional positioning options include having the patient supine with the head of the bed elevated 30° to 45° or the patient in the lateral decubitus position with the effusion side down, with needle placement in the mid-axillary line.
- Identify all surrounding structures including the lungs, diaphragm, and adjacent organs. The pleural effusion will most often be hypoechoic and can serve as a good acoustic window. It may appear more echogenic on ultrasonography depending on the protein content and amount of inflammatory cells present. Determine the borders of the fluid collection, and note the site of least obstructed access to the most amount of fluid (**Fig. 6**).
- Anesthetize the insertion site. Insert the needle over the superior aspect of the rib to avoid the neurovascular bundle. Keep the needle tip in the sonographic window as it is advanced. Maintain negative pressure on the syringe until fluid is withdrawn. A catheter may be placed using the Seldinger technique, and attaching a tubing set to a drainage bag or vacuum bottle (**Fig. 7**).[14]

Box 2
Supplies needed for thoracentesis

Sterile drapes or towels

Sterile ultrasound transducer cover with sterile ultrasound gel

Chlorhexidine or appropriate skin antiseptic

Lidocaine 1% or 2% with epinephrine

Injection needle (25 gauge, 1.5 inch)

Long 16- to 18-gauge needle (5–10 cm)

5-mL and 20-mL or 60-mL Luer-lock syringes

Three-way stopcock

Tubing set with aspiration adaptors

Specimen vials or blood tubes, drainage bag, or vacuum bottle

Central venous access kit or thoracentesis kit if a catheter will be left in place

No. 11 blade scalpel

Sterile gauze pads

Pearls and Pitfalls

- Although the risk of injuring solid organs is reduced using dynamic ultrasound guidance, the selected site of insertion should stay cephalad to the eighth intercostal space.
- Take note of changes in the position and depth of the effusion during the respiratory cycle. For this reason it is recommended that the entire thoracentesis be performed under dynamic ultrasound guidance rather than a static approach. Needle location can be confirmed in the pleural space by injecting a few milliliters of saline with visualization of bubbling within the pleural space.
- Although phased-array or curvilinear transducers are more commonly used, higher-frequency linear transducers may allow for better needle visualization.

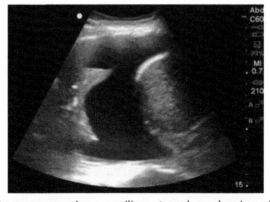

Fig. 6. Bedside ultrasonogram using a curvilinear transducer showing a large right pleural effusion over the liver. The lung parenchyma can be seen floating in the effusion on the left side of the image. Note that the entire hemidiaphragm is visualized on this view. (*Courtesy of* T. Wu, MD, Phoenix, AZ.)

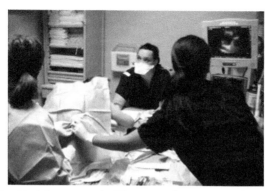

Fig. 7. Ultrasound-guided thoracentesis. (*Courtesy of* T. Wu, MD, Phoenix, AZ.)

The phased-array or curvilinear transducer should be used initially to identify the largest fluid collection with the least obstructed point of access, at which point a linear probe can be used to initiate the procedure.

- The long-axis view offers the advantage of the monitoring the entire trajectory of the needle throughout the procedure; however, limited windows within the intercostal space may make this approach more difficult.
- Dynamic ultrasound guidance offers the additional advantage of monitoring lung reexpansion as the effusion is drained. As the lung returns closer to the chest wall, it may be necessary to retract the needle to avoid inadvertent organ puncture.

ULTRASOUND-GUIDED PARACENTESIS
Background

Ascites has a broad spectrum of etiology. Approximately 80% to 85% of cases in the United States are secondary to parenchymal liver disease, most commonly alcoholic liver disease. Other causes include malignancy, heart failure, tuberculosis, malnutrition or protein-deficient states, pancreatic disease, or renal failure (dialysis ascites).

Paracentesis can be performed for both diagnostic and therapeutic purposes. Diagnostic analysis is most useful in new-onset ascites or in patients appearing ill in whom bacterial peritonitis is suspected. Patients requiring therapeutic paracentesis may present with cardiorespiratory compromise secondary to mass effect of tense ascites, and mechanical obstruction in patients who have otherwise failed diuretic therapy.

Ultrasonography has long been used to assist with paracentesis, owing to its ease of use and high success rate. In a 2005 study comparing ultrasound-guided with blinded paracentesis, 95% of the ultrasound group had a safe and successful aspiration while only 61% of those in the blinded group were successful.[15]

Diagnosis

Although small-volume ascites may be asymptomatic, the diagnosis by physical examination is generally straightforward in patients with any significant peritoneal fluid requiring therapeutic drainage. Findings that support the diagnosis include a shifting dullness or peripheral edema. Dullness does not manifest on physical examination until there is sufficient intraperitoneal fluid, usually greater than 1500 mL.[16] Shifting dullness has been shown in numerous studies to be an unreliable finding.

Ultrasonography is highly sensitive for diagnosing intra-abdominal fluid, and is able to detect as little as 100 mL of free fluid.[17] Improved resolution in newer ultrasound machines has given practitioners the ability to visualize even 5 to 10 mL of free fluid adjacent to the urinary bladder (**Fig. 8**).[18,19]

Precautions

- Do not perform a skin puncture through cellulitis, abscess, or other signs of superficial infection.
- There are no absolute contraindications to ultrasound-guided paracentesis, and it is generally a safe procedure with few significant complications despite the comorbid conditions present in these patients.
- Risks associated with paracentesis are greatly reduced with ultrasonography, including damage to the liver, spleen, gastrointestinal tract, urinary bladder, or abdominal vasculature.
- Many patients may have some degree of underlying coagulopathy or thrombocytopenia. Consider administration of blood products to patients with a prothrombin time greater than 20 seconds, international normalized ratio (INR) greater than 2.0, or a platelet count of less than 50,000/mm^3.[20,21] Some evidence shows this may not be necessary if using ultrasound guidance or if performed by experienced providers, with reports of platelet counts as low as 19,000/mm^3 or INR as high as 8.7 that require no product transfusion.[22,23]
- An abdominal wall hematoma is one of the more common complications encountered, but still only occurs in 1% to 2% of paracenteses despite more than 70% of patients having concurrent coagulopathy.[20] Other risks include postprocedural hypotension, hemoperitoneum, or electrolyte changes such as hyponatremia.

Procedure

- Supplies needed for paracentesis are listed in **Box 3**.
- The patient should have an empty urinary bladder. The patient is positioned supine with the head of the bed slightly elevated to take restrictive forces off of the diaphragm and to concentrate ascitic fluid into dependent portions of the peritoneal cavity.

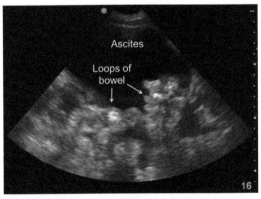

Fig. 8. Ultrasonogram of bowel floating in ascites as seen with a phased-array transducer. Note the depth markings on the right side of the image, showing greater than 5 cm of fluid between the peritoneal wall and loops of bowel. (*Courtesy of* T. Wu, MD, Phoenix, AZ.)

| Box 3 |
Supplies needed for paracentesis
Sterile drapes or towels
Sterile ultrasound transducer cover with sterile ultrasound gel
Chlorhexidine or appropriate skin antiseptic
Lidocaine 1% or 2% with epinephrine
Injection needle (25 gauge, 1.5 inch)
Paracentesis catheter or 18- to 22-gauge needle (1.5 or 3.5 inch)
5-mL, 10-mL, and 60-mL Luer-lock syringes
Tubing set with aspiration adaptors
Specimen vials or blood tubes, vacuum bottles
No. 11 blade scalpel
Tape or an adhesive bandage
Sterile gauze pads

- Use a 5- to 2-MHz curvilinear transducer or a 5- to 1-MHz phased-array transducer to visualize the peritoneal fluid and identify surrounding structures. When choosing a site of entry, avoid any local skin infection, collateral veins, or scar tissue.
- Most commonly, the bilateral lower quadrants provide reliable access to the ascitic fluid without interference from other structures. Ultrasonography can confirm placement lateral to the rectus sheath to avoid the inferior epigastric artery. The site is typically 5 cm cephalad and medial to the anterior superior iliac spine, although ultrasound will guide the provider to the largest pocket of peritoneal fluid where no bowel is immediately against the abdominal wall.
- After determining the best site of entry using bedside ultrasonography, prepare and drape the patient in the usual sterile fashion, including sterile preparation of the ultrasound transducer.
- Determine the trajectory of the needle using ultrasound guidance. Use of the Z-tract method is recommended to reduce the risk of postprocedural leak of ascitic fluid; this is accomplished by pulling the skin 2 cm downward with lateral traction before needle puncture. After penetrating the epidermis and dermis, release the tension on the skin and advance through underlying subcutaneous tissues and the peritoneum.
- Maintain negative pressure on the syringe with gentle aspiration while advancing the needle. Maintain the needle tip in the field of view at all times, by either long-axis or short long-axis views. Ensure the needle tip stays at a safe distance from intestinal loops (**Fig. 9**).
- If performing a diagnostic paracentesis, drainage of 200 mL of fluid is typically more than sufficient for evaluation. If performing a therapeutic paracentesis and large volumes are to be removed, a catheter may be placed over the needle using the Seldinger technique.

Pearls and Pitfalls

- Estimating the amount of fluid present by ultrasonographic appearance can be difficult and imprecise; however, a general rule is that for every 1 cm of visible fluid around intestinal loops, there is an estimated 1 L of ascitic fluid present.

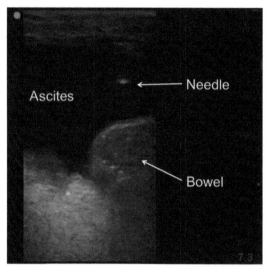

Fig. 9. Ultrasound-guided paracentesis. The hyperechoic needle is seen in the short axis, prohibiting visualization of the entire needle tract. (*Courtesy of* T. Wu, MD, Phoenix, AZ.)

- Opinions vary regarding needle diameter. If performing a diagnostic paracentesis, a 22-gauge needle may be more appropriate. If large-volume paracentesis is anticipated, it may be more appropriate to use a larger-diameter needle, such as an 18-gauge or larger, to allow a more timely removal of ascitic fluid.
- As the peritoneal cavity is decompressed, the needle or catheter tip may stop flowing and need repositioning, which can be done with ultrasound guidance. Injection of 3 to 5 mL of normal saline may clear any small obstruction in the catheter tubing and also help localize the catheter tip, as it is not as echogenic as a needle tip and may be difficult to identify on a sonogram.

ULTRASOUND-GUIDED LUMBAR PUNCTURE
Background

Headache and altered level of consciousness can be the presenting symptoms of several life-threatening conditions, such as bacterial meningitis or subarachnoid hemorrhage. Timely and accurate diagnosis is essential, and may often require emergent lumbar puncture (LP). Other less emergent indications for LP include idiopathic intracranial hypertension (formerly known as pseudotumor cerebri), demyelinating disorders, tertiary syphilis, and other inflammatory conditions of the central nervous system (CNS).

There is a continual cycling of cerebrospinal fluid (CSF) between its production by the choroid plexus and its absorption by the venous system. CSF flows continuously from the ventricles through the spinal canal with homogeneous cellular contents throughout, allowing for safe and accurate CSF sampling at the level of the cauda equina. The CNS of an average adult has approximately 140 mL of CSF, with 30 mL in the spinal canal. The average production rate of CSF is 0.35 mL/min, regenerating the amount lost during an average LP in less than an hour.[9]

LP has traditionally relied on palpable landmarks to identify the lower lumbar interspinous spaces. Ultrasound guidance has gained popularity, particularly in obese patients or those with distorted anatomy. By allowing for direct visualization of the targeted interspinous space, the number of unsuccessful attempts can be minimized.[24,25]

Diagnosis

Physical examination may assist in making the diagnosis of meningitis, particularly if the patient presents with characteristic findings of nuchal rigidity, Kernig or Brudzinski signs, or a petechial rash with fever. However, infectious conditions of the CSF cannot be excluded without direct fluid analysis.

A suspected subarachnoid hemorrhage (SAH) is another emergent indication for LP. Traditionally, noncontrast head CT with LP has been required to confirm or exclude the presence of SAH. If presenting within the first 24 hours of onset, diagnosis by CT alone is reported to have an accuracy of 95% to 98%; however, this quickly diminishes with time to 76% at 48 hours and 50% at 7 days.[9]

Precautions

- Relative contraindications exist for LP, particularly in those with elevated intracranial pressure or a space-occupying CNS lesion. Head CT is recommended before LP to minimize the risk of herniation, although it is an infrequent complication with only 22 case reports identified, and has been shown to occur in severe cases of bacterial meningitis without LP.[26]
- Injury to the dural or arachnoid vessels can occur, causing hemorrhage into the CSF. Though usually of little consequence, there is increased concern in those with active bacteremia, human immunodeficiency virus infection, or hemophilia. Spinal epidural hematomas are uncommon but may develop in those with a bleeding diathesis or thrombocytopenia, or in those who are otherwise coagulopathic. Spinal subdural hematomas are even less common.[27]
- There are no absolute guidelines. However, patients known to be anticoagulated, hemophiliac, or otherwise coagulopathic should consider having any deficiencies corrected before LP, although some studies have shown no adverse events in patients with platelet counts as low as $10,000/mm^3$.[28]

Procedure

- Supplies needed for LP are listed in **Box 4**
- If opening pressure is required, patient should lie in in a lateral decubitus position with the head and legs tucked toward the umbilicus for pressure measurement. Otherwise, the patient may be placed in a seated position, leaning forward, with the arms and head resting on a bedside table.
- A high-frequency 13- to 5-MHz linear array transducer is preferred. However, in patients with significant amounts of soft tissue a lower frequency curvilinear transducer may be required.
- Prepare and drape the patient in the usual sterile fashion, including sterile preparation of the ultrasound transducer.
- Start by placing the probe in a transverse fashion, perpendicular to the long axis of the patient's spine, along the midline of the spine, at the level of the iliac crests.
- Scan until a bright white hyperechoic spinous process is identified. It should case a large, far-field shadow. The spinous process will be visualized between the paraspinal musculature as seen in the transverse view. The midline of the patient is identified as the spinous process is centered in the middle of the ultrasound screen, which correlates directly with the middle of the probe (**Fig. 10**).
- Mark this location with a sterile marker on the patient to identify midline. Use ultrasound guidance to identify 2 additional spinous processes in a similar manner,

---

Box 4
Supplies needed for lumbar puncture

Sterile drapes or towels

Sterile ultrasound transducer cover with sterile ultrasound gel

Linear ultrasound transducer

Iodine or appropriate skin antiseptic

Lidocaine 1% or 2% with epinephrine

Injection needle (25 gauge, 1.5 inch)

3.5- to 5-inch spinal needle (18–22 gauge)

5-mL Luer-lock syringe

Manometer

Collection tubes

Sterile marker

Tape or adhesive bandage

Sterile gauze pads

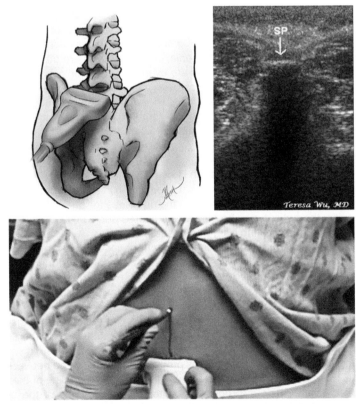

Fig. 10. Transverse views of the lumbar spine. These views identify the spinous processes (SP) at several lumbar levels, allowing for determination of the midline. (*Courtesy of* T. Wu, MD, Phoenix, AZ; and N. Hatch, MD, Phoenix, AZ.)

and mark these as well. This mapping provides a line that follows the long axis of the spine in the midline, and helps the provider identify any scoliosis of the spine.

- Next, rotate the transducer 90° so that it lies parallel to the long axis of the spine. Scan along the previously identified midline of the patient's back.
- As seen in the corresponding images, the spinous processes now appear as hyperechoic curves casting dark, far-field shadows, with interspinous spaces visualized between 2 adjacent spinous processes (**Fig. 11**).
- Scan along the long axis of the spine until the interspinous space is centered in the screen with a spinous process identified on either side. Use a sterile marker to draw a line at this spot perpendicular to the previous midline identified.
- The intersection of these 2 lines identifies the point of entry for the spinal needle (**Fig. 12**).

Pearls and Pitfalls

- Ultrasound-guided LPs can be performed in a static or dynamic fashion, although limited space and the need for a trained assistant makes real-time visualization difficult. Most commonly, ultrasonography is used to identify landmarks and mark proper needle placement, with the lumbar puncture then carried out in a traditional fashion.

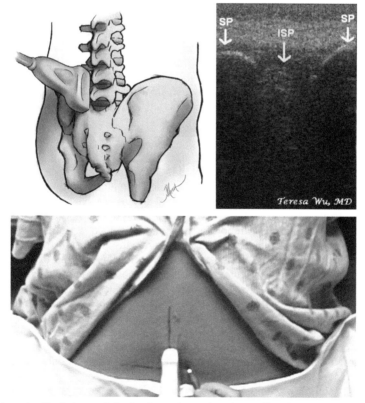

Fig. 11. Longitudinal views of the lumbar spine. After the midline has been identified, this view identifies the interspinous space (ISP) located between spinous processes (SP). (*Courtesy of* T. Wu, MD, Phoenix, AZ; and N. Hatch, MD, Phoenix, AZ.)

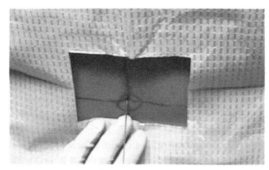

Fig. 12. Ultrasound mapping to identify the site of entry where the interspinous space is bisected along the midline. The lumbar puncture is then performed using the standard technique. (*Courtesy of* T. Wu, MD, Phoenix, AZ.)

- When attempting to visualize 2 adjacent spinous processes on the longitudinal view, start with your probe directly over the patient's midline. You may need to rotate the probe by just a few millimeters to align both spinous processes on the screen simultaneously.
- With longitudinal views it is imperative to stay directly over the midline. Any lateral deviation may bring transverse processes into view, which can be easily mistaken for spinous processes in 2-dimensional ultrasonography.
- Higher-resolution ultrasonography may have the capability to identify the ligamentum flavum within the interspinous space just superficial to the epidural space. It appears as a bright, white, hyperechoic structure deep to the level of the spinous processes. Ultrasonographic identification of this structure can provide an estimate of the distance between skin and the spinal canal before needle insertion.

ULTRASOUND-GUIDED NERVE BLOCKS
Background

Regional anesthesia offers many advantages in patients with multisystem trauma, those who are critically ill, or those who have pain from an isolated region that would otherwise require procedural sedation or general anesthesia. Nerve blocks are generally better tolerated than direct infiltration of the injured site, and often require less infused anesthetic volume. Common indications for regional anesthesia include the reduction of fractures and dislocations, abscess drainage, laceration repair, minor surgical procedures, or for comfort measures in patients with localized trauma.[29–31]

Traditional regional anesthesia techniques have relied on anatomic landmarks and nerve stimulators; however, the introduction of ultrasound guidance has improved successful anesthetic infiltration and a reduction in injury to surrounding structures.[29,30,32] Multiple studies have shown superiority of ultrasound-guided nerve blocks, with an average success rate of 95% compared with 70% to 85% using landmarks and nerve stimulation alone. Other proven benefits include significantly faster times to nerve blockade, reduced complications, and smaller doses of anesthetic required.[18,33]

The most common sites for ultrasound-guided regional anesthesia include the brachial plexus, intercostal nerves, and peripheral nerves such as the radial, median, ulnar, femoral, sciatic, popliteal, and saphenous nerves. Multiple different approaches are possible for a given nerve, such as the brachial plexus, where there are well-described techniques for supraclavicular, intraclavicular, interscalene, and axillary approaches.

Regional anesthesia is relatively straightforward in principle; however, the need for precision and understanding of complex anatomic relationships has kept it from being widely adapted across multiple specialties. Ultrasonography has made many of these procedures more accessible. The following serves as an introduction to regional anesthesia with several commonly used blocks described, although it is far from being a comprehensive review, and the reader should not consider it as such.

Precautions

- Particularly in the setting of a traumatized extremity, ensure that there is no evidence of compartment syndrome before starting the procedure. Although anesthesia may be important for patient comfort, it may mask important signs of a heralding compartment syndrome.
- Do not enter the skin through any areas of contaminated wounds, cellulitis, abscess, or rash.
- Use clinical judgment when considering the risks versus benefits when performing this procedure, particularly on patients with underlying coagulopathy. Long-acting anesthetics may also limit the physical examination of specialists if needed in a timely fashion.
- Risks associated with the procedure include damage of nerves, ineffective anesthesia, vascular infiltration, vascular disruption, hematoma formation, and local or systemic reactions to the anesthetic. Nerve damage is a reported complication thought to be secondary to intraneural sheath injection, a risk that is reduced by real-time ultrasonography. Perform and document a thorough neurologic examination before the procedure.
- Correct anatomic knowledge is essential for performing the block successfully and for avoiding complications. Several sites may have inherent risks attributable to specific adjacent structures, such as brachial plexus blocks and the associated risk for pneumothorax, spinal cord injury, and phrenic nerve damage.

Procedure

- Supplies needed for regional nerve block are listed in **Box 5**.
- The patient should be placed in a position of comfort that allows unobstructed access to the region of interest.
- The patient should be in a closely monitored setting on a cardiopulmonary monitor as the block is performed, and should be watched carefully for at least 15 to 30 minutes following the procedure.
- A high-frequency linear-array transducer (15–10 MHz) is preferred. However, deeper structures may be better visualized using a lower-frequency curvilinear transducer.
- After visualizing the nerve bundle and determining the best site of entry using bedside ultrasonography, prepare and drape the patient in the usual fashion, including sterile preparation of the ultrasound transducer. Apply a generous amount of sterile gel to the site.
- The needle should be attached to the syringe indirectly using extension tubing. The provider performing the block should have one hand stabilizing the needle while advancing it with the other hand, meanwhile using the transducer for dynamic ultrasound guidance. An assistant should be available to hold the syringe, aspirate fluid, and inject fluid when appropriate.

Box 5
Supplies needed for regional nerve block

Sterile drapes or towels

Sterile ultrasound transducer cover with sterile ultrasound gel

Linear ultrasound transducer

Chlorhexidine or appropriate skin antiseptic

Lidocaine 1% or 2% with epinephrine

Long-acting local anesthetic

Injection needle (25 gauge, 1.5 inch)

Noncutting injection 22- to 24-gauge needle (spinal needle)

5-mL and 20-mL Luer-lock syringes

Short extension tubing set

Sterile marker

Tape and gauze

Sterile gauze pads

- For better visualization of the nerve fibers turn down the overall gain, focusing on the hyperechoic nerve tissue and making the adjacent muscle bellies dim and dark. Nerves for regional anesthesia will usually be found between muscular junctions in distinct planes within the intermuscular space.
- Place the transducer in a transverse plane to obtain a cross-sectional view of the target nerves. Proximally, at the level of the cervical roots, nerves have a monofascicular appearance when viewed in cross section. As the nerves course distally, the bundle adopts a honeycomb appearance as the hyperechoic connective tissue (epineurium and perineurium) surrounds hypoechoic nerve bundles.[34,35]
- Once the target nerve is identified, center it in the screen and rotate the transducer to obtain longitudinal views of the nerve. It should maintain its unique echotexture of hyperechoic connective tissue surrounding individual hypoechoic fascicle groups.
- Infiltrate superficial tissues with a small amount of local anesthetic to maximize patient comfort and cooperation.
- Under direct ultrasonographic visualization, insert the needle and aim its tip at the target nerve. Keep the needle bevel perpendicular to the transducer to maximize echogenicity. Maintain negative pressure by gently aspirating on the syringe while advancing, to ensure no vessel is entered before infiltration (**Fig. 13**).
- When the needle is in the desired location, test by injecting a 1- to 2-mL aliquot of anesthetic, which should confirm needle-tip location, creating an anechoic pocket that surrounds the nerve bundle.

Femoral Nerve Block

- Blockade of the femoral nerve provides anesthesia to the femur, anterior thigh, and knee. As it leaves the lumbar plexus it courses distally between the iliacus and psoas major muscle bodies. As it reaches the proximal thigh it passes beneath the inguinal ligament, midway between the anterior superior iliac spine and the pubic tubercle, where it then lies anterior to the iliopsoas muscle and lateral to the femoral artery.

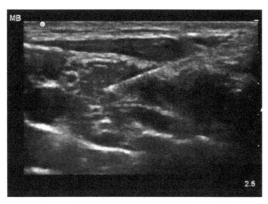

Fig. 13. Ultrasound-guided nerve block. Note the trajectory of the needle seen in its long axis as it comes into contact with a peripheral nerve seen in its short axis. (*Courtesy of* T. Wu, MD, Phoenix, AZ.)

- Multiple fascial planes are found in the region of the femoral sheath, although all may not be readily visible. The fascia lata covers the muscles of the hip flexors and quadriceps. The femoral vessels are contained within a thick, fibrous sheath. The femoral nerve lies outside this sheath in a separate tissue plane, beneath the fascia iliaca (**Figs. 14** and **15**). Failure to penetrate the fascia iliaca will manifest as perivascular anesthetic deposition, although it will not reach the adjacent femoral nerve.
- A 3-in-1 femoral nerve block is useful for proximal thigh or hip injuries. This block includes additional blockade of the lateral femoral cutaneous and obturator nerves, which provide sensation to the lateral and medial thighs, respectively. All 3 nerves lie beneath the fascia iliaca. It is performed in the same manner as

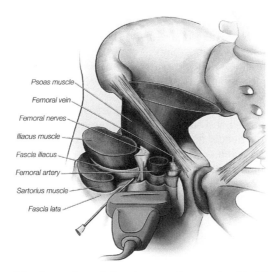

Fig. 14. Anatomy of the femoral canal showing an ultrasound-guided femoral nerve block. The femoral nerve is located beneath the fascia iliacus and is separated from the adjacent femoral vessels. (*Courtesy of* N. Hatch, MD, Phoenix, AZ.)

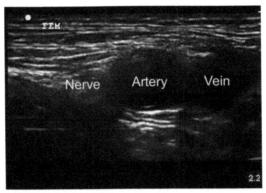

Fig. 15. Ultrasonographic appearance of the femoral canal anatomy in a transverse view. (*Courtesy of* T. Wu, MD, Phoenix, AZ.)

a femoral block, with a larger volume of anesthetic infiltrated around the femoral nerve (20–30 mL) while maintaining firm pressure several centimeters distal to the needle-insertion site to prevent distal spread.[36]

Pearls and Pitfalls

- Minimize complications by identifying all adjacent vascular and critical structures that should be avoided. The importance of understanding anatomy in the region of interest, as well as potential complications, cannot be overemphasized.
- The appearance of nerves in cross section on ultrasonography can be easily confused with tendons and lymph nodes. Trace the structure of interest along its axis. Lymph nodes are small and discrete, without continuation longer than several centimeters. Tendons will eventually transition into muscle, whereas nerves maintain their structure along the periphery of the muscle planes.
- Peripheral nerves are not inherently fixed to the structures that surround them, and may appear relatively mobile on ultrasonography. Nerves will not generally compress under the ultrasound transducer.
- The shape and echotexture of a nerve in short axis may vary, depending on the nerve and location. Shapes vary from round to triangular, depending on surrounding structures. The honeycomb appearance may not be as well pronounced in some nerves, particularly at more proximal sites, where many nerves may have a monofascicular appearance.
- Although the procedure may be accomplished with a variety of needles, the risk of damage to nerves and surrounding structures may be decreased by using a noncutting spinal needle as opposed to the standard cutting needles used for most other procedures.
- If the advancement of the needle elicits paresthesias, the needle tip should be withdrawn 1 to 2 mm so as to avoid the risk of intraneural injection. Be cautious of high pressures needed for infiltration or intense pain elicited, as these findings may signify intraneural injection.

ULTRASOUND-GUIDED PERITONSILLAR ABSCESS DRAINAGE
Background

Peritonsillar abscess (PTA) is a common deep-space infection of the head and neck that develops between the tonsillar capsule and the superior constrictor and palatopharyngeus muscles. If not properly identified and treated, it can progress to airway compromise and obstruction. Organisms are typically polymicrobial and often include anaerobes, *Staphylococcus*, *Streptococcus*, *Eikenella*, and *Haemophilus*.

Physical examination alone cannot reliably differentiate peritonsillar cellulitis from PTA, with blind aspirations resulting in greater than 12% false-negative rates. Ultrasonography offers immediate confirmation at the bedside, precise localization of the abscess before drainage, and the ability to keep the patient upright and in a position of comfort during the procedure.

Diagnosis

Standard imaging with CT for diagnosing PTA has sensitivity of 100% and specificity of 75%, whereas ultrasonography has sensitivity of 89% and specificity of 100%.[37] The anatomy of the peritonsillar region is complex. Use of an intracavitary transducer helps to identify surrounding anatomy and multiple key structures, the most important of which are the palatine tonsil and the internal carotid artery.

Precautions

- Failure to properly diagnose an abscess may lead to delayed intervention, with subsequent risk to the airway or abscess communication with other adjacent structures.
- Drainage of an abscess cavity may lead to spread of infectious contents with subsequent rupture, retropharyngeal abscess, or mediastinitis.
- Risks with drainage of a PTA are most notable for damage to surrounding structures, in particular the carotid artery, usually located within 5 to 25 mm of the abscess.

Procedure

- Supplies needed for PTA drainage are listed in **Box 6**.
- Use a high-frequency intracavitary transducer to visualize the peritonsillar space. Allowing patients to insert the probe themselves may make the procedure more tolerable and minimize the gag reflex. Once in place, guide the transducer face over the peritonsillar region.
- Thoroughly evaluate the peritonsillar space for abscess formation and multiple pockets, and identify the largest collection(s) most amenable to drainage (**Fig. 16**).
- Visualize the carotid artery, located posterolateral to the palatine tonsil and approximately 2.5 cm deep to the mucosal surface. It is best seen in the

---

Box 6
Supplies needed for peritonsillar abscess drainage

Intracavitary transducer cover with sterile ultrasound gel

Intracavitary ultrasound transducer

Topical and/or nebulized 4% lidocaine

18- to 20-gauge spinal needle with plastic cover (3.5–5 inch)

5-mL and 10-mL Luer-lock syringes

Bedside oral suction device

Airway equipment including a Macintosh blade

No. 11 blade scalpel

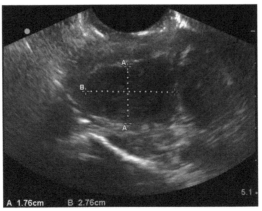

Fig. 16. A 1.76 × 2.76-cm peritonsillar abscess in the transverse plane. (*Courtesy of* T. Wu, MD, Phoenix, AZ.)

transverse plane. Define the relationship of the abscess pocket to the vessel, while mapping out the needle trajectory in the transverse plane so as to minimize risk of accidental arterial puncture.

- Use the depth markers on the right side of the ultrasound screen to note the depth of the abscess pocket and the depth of the carotid artery (**Fig. 17**).
- The carotid artery can be protected from inadvertent puncture by preparing the spinal needle before aspiration attempts. Remove the plastic needle guard, and cut 1 to 2 cm from its tip. Then reapply it around the needle. This action exposes a portion of the needle for the aspiration, but limits the depth to which it can be inserted.

Pearls and Pitfalls

- Adequate and safe drainage of a PTA requires an awake and cooperative patient. Plan the procedure, create a calm environment, and prepare the patient accordingly. When discussing the procedure with the patient, always refer to the transducer as the intracavitary rather than the transvaginal probe.

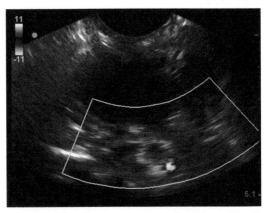

Fig. 17. Evaluation of peritonsillar abscess using color Doppler to identify the carotid artery. (*Courtesy of* T. Wu, MD, Phoenix, AZ.)

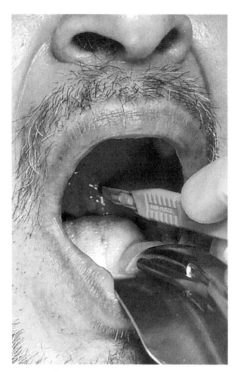

Fig. 18. Incision and drainage of a peritonsillar abscess following ultrasound localization at the bedside. (*Courtesy of* T. Wu, MD, Phoenix, AZ.)

- The appearance of a PTA can vary depending on the composition of the fluid, leading to some abscesses being overlooked even when using ultrasound guidance. Look for an echogenic, fluid-filled region creating a mass effect on the tonsil. If unsure of findings, anatomy, or orientation, it may be beneficial to compare with the contralateral side.
- Although the preferred method of aspiration is under dynamic ultrasound guidance, limited space and the presence of trismus may make simultaneous intraoral placement of the transducer and the drainage needle difficult. In these cases, use ultrasonography to confirm the presence of an abscess, noting its size, location, and depth. The aspiration or incision and drainage can then be performed after removing the transducer from the patient's oropharynx (**Fig. 18**).

SUMMARY

Ultrasound guidance can be used for a variety of procedures that have been traditionally performed using physical examination findings and anatomic landmark guidance alone. Using ultrasound guidance at the bedside minimizes risk and maximizes the chances of a successful procedure.

REFERENCES

1. Tirado A, Wu T, Noble VE, et al. Ultrasound-guided procedures in the emergency department—diagnostic and therapeutic asset. Emerg Med Clin North Am 2013; 31(1):117–49.

2. Tsang T, Enriquez-Sarano M, Freeman W, et al. 1127 consecutive therapeutic echocardiographically guided pericardiocenteses: clinical profile, practice patterns, and outcomes spanning 21 years. Mayo Clin Proc 2002;77:429.
3. Little W, Freeman G. Pericardial disease. Circulation 2006;113:1622.
4. Sagristà-Sauleda J, Angel J, Sambola A, et al. Hemodynamic effects of volume expansion in patients with cardiac tamponade. Circulation 2008;117:1545.
5. Pepi M, Muratori M. Echocardiography in the diagnosis and management of pericardial disease. J Cardiovasc Med (Hagerstown) 2006;7(7):533–44.
6. Vayre F, Lardoux H, Pezzano M, et al. Subxiphoid pericardiocentesis guided by contrast two-dimensional echocardiography in cardiac tamponade: experience of 110 consecutive patients. Eur J Echocardiogr 2000;1(1):66–71.
7. Tsang T, Freeman W, Barnes M, et al. Rescue echocardiographically guided pericardiocentesis for cardiac perforation complicating catheter-based procedures. The Mayo Clinical Experience. J Am Coll Cardiol 1998;32(5):1345–50.
8. Ozer H, Davutoglu V, Cakici M, et al. Echocardiography-guided pericardiocentesis with the apical approach. Turk Kardiyol Dern Ars 2009;37(3):177–81 [in Turkish].
9. Maisch B, Seferovic P, Ristic A, et al. Guidelines on the diagnosis and management of pericardial diseases executive summary; the task force on the diagnosis and management of pericardial diseases of the European Society of Cardiology. Eur Heart J 2004;25:587.
10. Roberts J, Hedges J. Clinical procedures in emergency medicine. Philadelphia: WB Saunders; 2004. p. 171–86, 305–22, 552–90, 841–59, 1197–222, 1371–92.
11. Rozycki G, Pennington S, Feliciano D. Surgeon-performed ultrasound in the critical care setting: its use as an extension of the physical examination to detect pleural effusion. J Trauma 2001;50(4):636–42.
12. Jones P, Moyers J, Rogers J. Ultrasound-guided thoracentesis: is it a safer method? Chest 2004;123(2):418–23.
13. Josephson T, Nordenskjold C, Larsson J, et al. Amount drained at ultrasound-guided thoracentesis and risk of pneumothorax. Acta Radiol 2009;50(1):42–7.
14. Liu Y, Lin Y, Liang S, et al. Ultrasound-guided pigtail catheters for drainage of various pleural diseases. Am J Emerg Med 2010;28(8):915–21.
15. Nazeer S, Dewbre H, Miller A. Ultrasound-assisted paracentesis performed by emergency physicians vs. the traditional technique: a prospective, randomized study. Am J Emerg Med 2005;23(3):363–7.
16. Cattau E, Benjamin S, Knuff T, et al. The accuracy of the physical exam in the diagnosis of suspected ascites. JAMA 1982;247:1164–6.
17. Runyon B. Management of adult patients with ascites caused by cirrhosis. Hepatology 2004;39:841–56.
18. Von Kuenssberg J, Stiller G, Wagner D. Sensitivity in detecting free intraperitoneal fluid with the pelvic views of the FAST exam. Am J Emerg Med 2003;21(6):476–8.
19. Ma O, Mateer J. Emergency ultrasound. New York: McGraw Hill; 2008. p. 449–62, 495–552.
20. Mallory A, Schaefer J. Complications of diagnostic paracentesis in patients with liver disease. JAMA 1978;239:628.
21. Runyon B. Paracentesis of ascitic fluid. A safe procedure. Arch Intern Med 1986;146(11):2259–61.
22. Lin C, Shih F, Ma M, et al. Should bleeding tendency deter abdominal paracentesis. Dig Liver Dis 2005;37(12):946–51.

23. Grabau C, Crago S, Hoff L, et al. Performance standards for therapeutic abdominal paracentesis. Hepatology 2004;40(2):484–8.
24. Strony R. Ultrasound-assisted lumbar puncture in obese patients. Crit Care Clin 2010;26(4):661–4.
25. Nomura J, Leech S, Shenbagamurthi S, et al. A randomized controlled trial of ultrasound-assisted lumbar puncture. J Ultrasound Med 2007;26(10):1341–8.
26. Joffe A. Lumbar puncture and brain herniation in acute bacterial meningitis: a review. J Intensive Care Med 2007;22:194.
27. Egede L, Moses H, Wang H. Spinal subdural hematoma: a rare complication of lumbar puncture. Md Med J 1999;48:15.
28. Howard S, Gajjar A, Ribeiro R, et al. Safety of lumbar puncture for children with acute lymphoblastic leukemia and thrombocytopenia. JAMA 2000;284:2222.
29. Abrahams M, Horn J, Noles L, et al. Evidence-based medicine: ultrasound guidance for truncal blocks. Reg Anesth Pain Med 2010;35(2):S36–42.
30. Walker K, McGrattan K, Aas-Eng K, et al. Ultrasound guidance for peripheral nerve blockade. Cochrane Database Syst Rev 2009;(4):CD006459.
31. Shah M, Blackmore M. The role of ultrasound in regional anesthesia. Br J Hosp Med 2010;71(12):718–27.
32. Orebaugh S, Williams B, Vallejo M, et al. Adverse outcomes associated with stimulator-based peripheral nerve blocks with versus without ultrasound visualization. Reg Anesth Pain Med 2009;34(3):251–5.
33. Grau T. Ultrasonography in the current practice of regional anaesthesia. Best Pract Res Clin Anaesthesiol 2005;19(2):175–200.
34. Bianchi S, Martinoli C. Ultrasound of the musculoskeletal system. New York: Springer Berlin Heidelberg; 2007. p. 97–103.
35. Beekman R, Visser L. High resolution sonography of the peripheral nervous system: a review of the literature. Eur J Neurol 2004;11:305–14.
36. Marhofer P, Kapral S, Sala-Blanch X. Three-in-one block. In: Hadzic A, editor. Textbook of regional anesthesia. New York: McGraw-Hill; 2007. p. 513.
37. Haeggstrom A, Gustafsson O, Engquist S, et al. Intraoral ultrasonography in the diagnosis of peritonsillar abscess. Otolaryngol Head Neck Surg 1993;108(3):243–7.

Index

Note: Page numbers of article titles are in **boldface** type.

A

Abscess(es)
  localization of
    for incision and drainage
      ultrasound-guided, 288–290
  musculoskeletal
    sonographic appearance of, 256
  periorbital
    ocular ultrasound for, 239–240
  tubo-ovarian
    bedside ultrasonography in, 221–222
Aneurysm(s)
  peripheral artery
    diagnostic ultrasonography for, 194–198
Ankle
  ultrasound-guided arthrocentesis for, 295–296
Arterial access
  ultrasound-guided, 284–287
Arterial occlusion
  of extremities
    diagnostic ultrasonography for, 200–205
Arthrocentesis
  ultrasound-guided, **293–301**
    anatomic sites, 294–299
      ankle, 295–296
      elbow, 298–299
      hip, 294–295
      knee, 294
      shoulder, 296–298
    clinical indications for, 293–294
    technique, 299–300
  visualizing the needle, 276–277
  vs. ultrasound-assisted procedures, 276
Artifact(s)
  on musculoskeletal ultrasonography, 253–254

B

β-HCG levels. *See* β-human chorionic gonadotropin (β-HCG) levels
β-human chorionic gonadotropin (β-HCG) levels
  in bedside ultrasonography for obstetric and gynecologic emergencies, 214

Crit Care Clin 30 (2014) 331–340
http://dx.doi.org/10.1016/S0749-0704(14)00010-4
0749-0704/14/$ – see front matter © 2014 Elsevier Inc. All rights reserved.

criticalcare.theclinics.com

Moving?

Make sure your subscription moves with you!

To notify us of your new address, find your **Clinics Account Number** (located on your mailing label above your name), and contact customer service at:

Email: journalscustomerservice-usa@elsevier.com

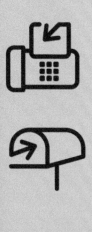

800-654-2452 (subscribers in the U.S. & Canada)
314-447-8871 (subscribers outside of the U.S. & Canada)

Fax number: 314-447-8029

Elsevier Health Sciences Division
Subscription Customer Service
3251 Riverport Lane
Maryland Heights, MO 63043

*To ensure uninterrupted delivery of your subscription, please notify us at least 4 weeks in advance of move.

Printed and bound by CPI Group (UK) Ltd, Croydon, CR0 4YY

03/10/2024

01040487-0015